An Extraordinary Life

A memoir by Cathy Rose

... and so, we danced in the early hours of the morning with the bedpan full of that beautiful, clear wee...

Stories of the joy of a makeshift emergency caesarean section birth are what make my grandmother's life the spectacular journey it is.
Having grown up hearing these unbelievable tales around the dinner table, I am thrilled that others can now experience them too.

84 years, 7 languages, 35 countries & counting...

A life so spectacular deserves a true and lasting record, and I am honoured to be a part of it.

Monique S. Rose

MY CHILDHOOD

How different things were in the 1930s. If you happened to be born into a poor family, you learned very early that you would not always have what you might want.

Unlike today's children with all the toys and gadgets available to them. We would be happy with a ball or a colouring book as the only gift for a birthday. It was safe to play out on the street with the neighbourhood children. We would play hopscotch or hide and seek for hours.

Our house was too small to play inside so even when it was cold in winter we would be outside until it got dark, which in winter was as early as 4:30 pm. I did not like the winters much. Except when it was so cold that the lakes and rivers froze to ice, and made a path so that I could skate to and from school. I love ice skating and could skate at the age of five years old. People used to call me Sonja Henie after a famous Dutch skater, so I am told.

I remember some pretty special treats in the summer holidays. We were allowed to hire a bicycle for a few days and took turns learning to ride it. Only much later, when I went to high school did I get my own bike. Always second hand of course.

The other treat in the summer holidays was when the older boys were allowed to hire a rowing boat for a few days. Now this was really special. I did not want to miss a minute and took my bucket of potatoes with me in the boat. That was my job in the holidays. I was to peel a bucket full of potatoes every day. I thought that was such fun, to sit and peel the potatoes while being rowed along by my brothers. My older sister Riet was not so lucky, she had to help mum at home and only got a turn once the housework was done. Though, she never seemed to mind.

There were ten of us, and I was a middle child. Number six in fact. Now thinking back, I find it quite strange that the boys never had to help out with anything. No wonder my mother almost had a nervous breakdown after the fourth boy was born. Only then did my father start to help her. He would make the beds and peel the potatoes at night for the next day.

I was seven years old when the war broke out. I remember the bombing of Schiphol, the nearby airport. The fighting only lasted five days as the small Dutch army was no match for the invading Germans. I was very scared our house would be hit, and we all hid in mum and dad's bed during the bombardments.

Life changed dramatically as the German army took charge. All able young men were taken to Germany to work there. Many went underground and formed a powerful resistance army. They saved many British pilots when their plane got shot down flying over to bomb Germany. My brothers were still too young and my dad just a bit too old, so none of my family had to go underground or to Germany. We were very grateful for that.

At night we were not allowed to show any light, so windows had to be covered with black paper. The German soldiers lived amongst us in houses they had confiscated, and they did not want the British planes to know where they were.

Food was rationed. At first, there was still enough, but as time went on and we were feeding the German army as well as sending food to Germany, things got much worse. The whole economy was suffering. Heating was a coal stove, but even coal was running out. After four years of war, things were getting desperate.

Shops were empty. Amsterdam was quickly running out of food. The black market was doing a roaring trade, but poor people could not afford the ridiculously high prices. The only food we could still get were sugar beets. We ate them for breakfast, lunch and dinner. The winter of 1944-45 was a winter I will never forget. It was bitterly cold. Nothing was fun anymore; when you are hungry and cold and you don't have enough warm blankets or clothes. I used to love ice skating, but this winter I told my friends, "I won't come as I get too hungry". People were dying in the streets.

There were some well-to-do people in our church. One of the chaplains liaised with these families, and they agreed to have a child from a poor family have a meal once a day with them. Two of my brothers were picked. Every afternoon they went to get a decent plate of dinner. The rest of us went to the school soup kitchen. The German's gave us their potato skins which were boiled up and given to us as soup. Of course, there was very little nutrition in it, but better something than nothing.

One blessed day, Chaplain Sul came and told my mother he had found another family willing to feed a child. He thought it should be Riet as she looked the skinniest. Riet was very shy, and although hungry, she did not want to go by herself. As the offer was only for one child, the priest asked if I wanted to go. Yes of course! I was only too happy to go. So every day at 12:30 I walked the half hour so the Sormani family. They must have decided that I would be more comfortable eating by myself. Although they were very kind people, it was here that I felt for the first time that I came from a poor family.

I would wear the same clothes every day and may not have smelled very nice. They were of a different social standing.

My brother Ben went to the Van Toorens. Their children went to the same school as us. Johan was in Ben's class, and they became good friends.

Louis went to the Sloothaaks, who owned the local garage. One day after finishing his meal, Louis decided to go to the school soup kitchen. When you are a fourteen-year-old growing teenager, one plate of food is not necessarily filling you up. But never having been truly hungry, one may not understand that. Anyway, Mr Sloothaak saw Louis going to the soup kitchen and was furious. He came to see my mum and told her that Louis was greedy, and he did not want to see him anymore. We were all so embarrassed for him. I think Mum even tried to tell Mr Sloothaak that Louis went to the soup kitchen to give his portion to his brother, even if that may not have been true. But to no avail. Louis had lost his chance, and they did not want to see him anymore. Poor Louis, we all felt terrible for him.

We only went to school half days now and the afternoons were filled with hunting for food. The Germans always had trucks passing with potatoes and beans, and we found that they dropped the odd potato or bean in the snow. The Amsterdam forest had some fields, and as we were always playing there, we once found a potato in the ground. So we started digging around and found quite a few potatoes. We took them home, and my surprised mum asked, "where did you find them?" We told her, "in the field." She said, "just don't tell anybody about this." She knew they were seed potatoes the Germans had planted. What a beautiful meal we had that night!

There was only one farm in the Amsterdam forest. The farmer was a member of our church. We were allowed to fetch five litres of milk once a week. They were the Van Duynhovens. My younger brother Fons spent a lot of time on their farm even after the war, and ended up marrying one of the daughters, Nel. First, he migrated to Canada at the age of twenty-one, then he returned to Holland to marry Nel, and she went to Canada to live there with him. They are still there these days and have a large family of five sons and twelve grandchildren.

It must have been so hard for my parents during those war years, raising ten children without ever having enough food or clothing. We had an old wood furnace to cook on, though wood was scarce, and I remember my Dad going out at night with the two eldest boys to cut down a tree somewhere. The trees in the Kalfjes laan, which is on the border of Buitenveldert and Nieuwer Amstel, were slowly disappearing. Clothes were scarce too. We all wore clogs (wooden shoes). Imagine not having any soap or soap powder for the washing! First we still had green soap, but when that was not available anymore, we used clay soap. I don't know what that was made of, but it did not clean well. Two of my brothers were bed wetters. How do you wash pyjamas and sheets without soap?

We were scared of the Germans, but not all of them were bad people. Indoctrinated in their youth, they just followed orders, and most of them had no idea what was going on back in Germany. They got the orders to raid the Jewish quarters and one day my aunty who had a Jewish neighbour and lived in the Jewish quarter told my parents that her neighbour Mrs Wouk had been picked up that night. She would have been put on a train with thousands of other Jews and taken to Germany to a concentration camp and eventually to the gas chambers. We only learned later what went on there.

Some Dutch people hid their Jewish friends in their homes, but if they were found out, they too were transported to the concentration camp. If they were useful to the Germans, they were not killed but forced to do the most atrocious things. After the War, they told us their stories, which I won't recount as it is too distressing. It is unbelievable how people can do such things to other people. Most soldiers who lived close to us did not know about this.

A German soldier once gave me a beautiful doll. When my mother went to ask him why he had given me the doll, he said he had a little girl my age and did not think he would ever see her again. I was not a 'dolly' girl and gave the doll to my sister Riet.

I was twelve years old when Amsterdam was liberated at last by the allied soldiers. All school children were allowed to stand on the roof of our school to wave at the aeroplanes of our liberators. What joy!! The Swedish people sent thousands of loaves of beautiful white bread. Each person got half a loaf, so our family got six loaves, and do you know what my Dad did? He called us all around the table and said "You can all eat your half a loaf," and he cut the loaves in half. Just fresh bread, as we did not have anything on it yet, but that bread tasted so incredibly good!! The youngest ones could not finish it, and the older ones were quick to beg for the rest, but my dad quickly stopped that. "No, they can keep it 'til later. Everyone can do with it what they want. Eat it all now, or save it for later". Things improved quickly from there. We were sent food from the Scandinavian countries, especially Sweden, and from the USA. We were also sent a lot of clothes - sure it was second hand, but to it us it was like Christmas when a huge box full of clothes was delivered. I remember there were coats, dresses, jumpers, pants, skirts, socks and shoes. We all got something as there were all sizes. I was lucky to get a very nice woollen dress and a warm coat, and I felt I looked a million dollars in my new coat.

There were food parcels delivered at Schiphol airport. One of the neighbours worked at the airport and when a package got broken, the contents were shared among the workers. Now, this neighbour had seven children himself, but when he brought something home, he would share whatever he got with all the neighbours. Sometimes it would be a little bit of tea or some chocolate. Not much and he could easily have kept it for his own family, but he chose to share it as we were still short of everything for months. One thing we were given very soon were nutritious biscuits. They came in a large tin of about twenty kilograms. They stilled our hunger in those first weeks.

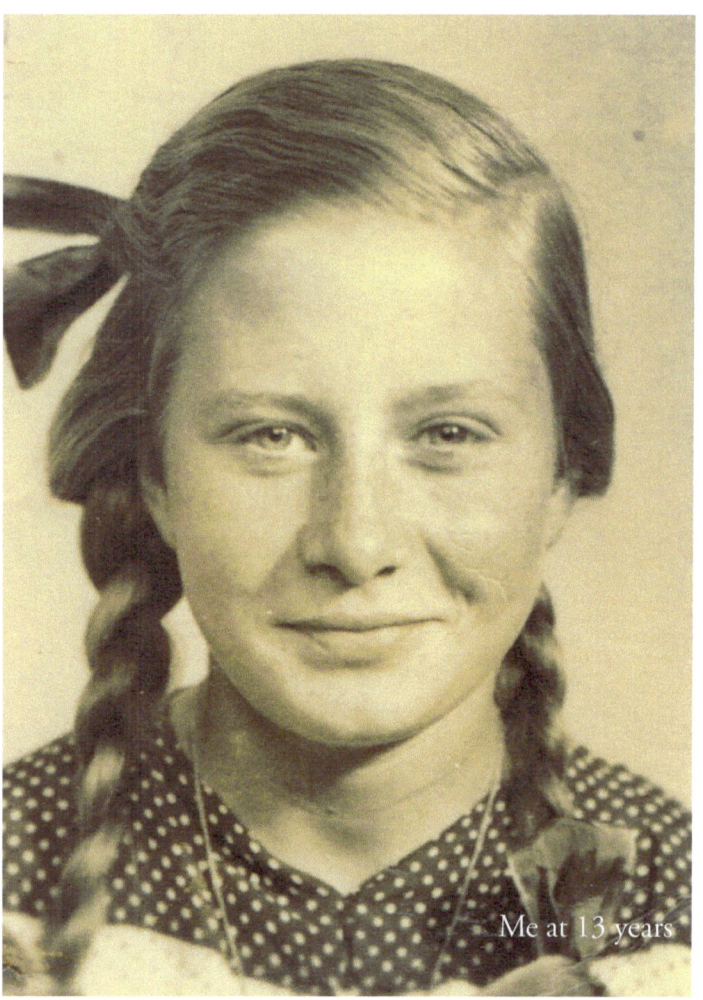

Me at 13 years

We soon found a use for the empty tins. Living on the water we could make a boat from fifteen tins by tying the tops together with fencing wire. We would tie four rows of three tin together and then one long piece around all the tins to hold them together. We could make boats that up to three kids could sit on if we used eighteen tins. None of us could swim but there was never an accident, and we had a lot of fun with our rafts. Life started to get better with each passing day.

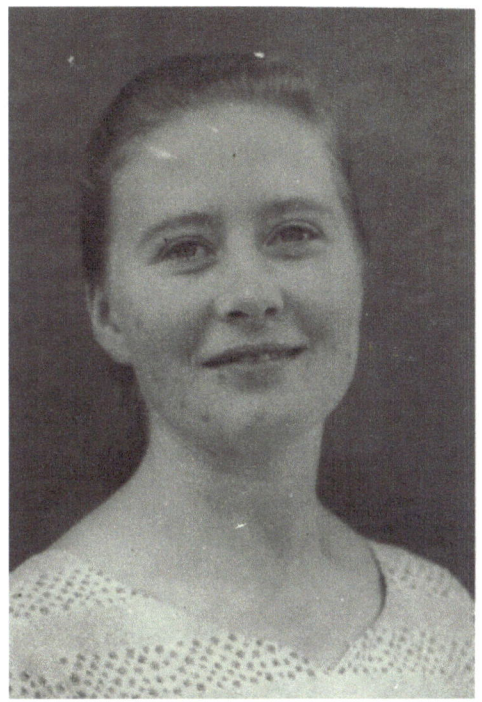

Me at 21 years

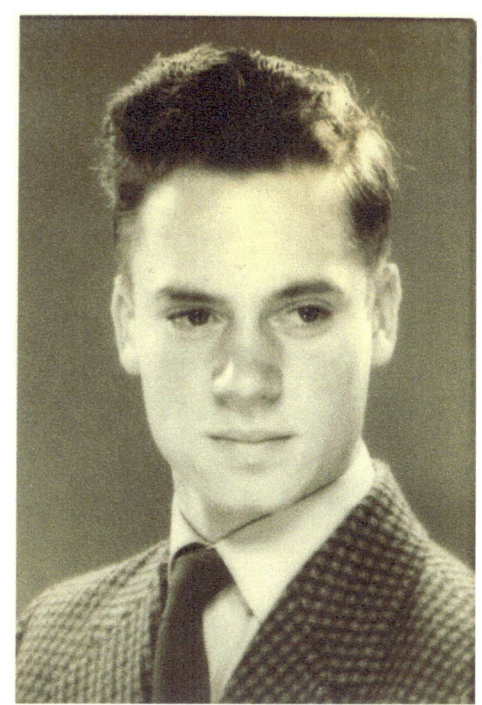

Faas, my youngest brother

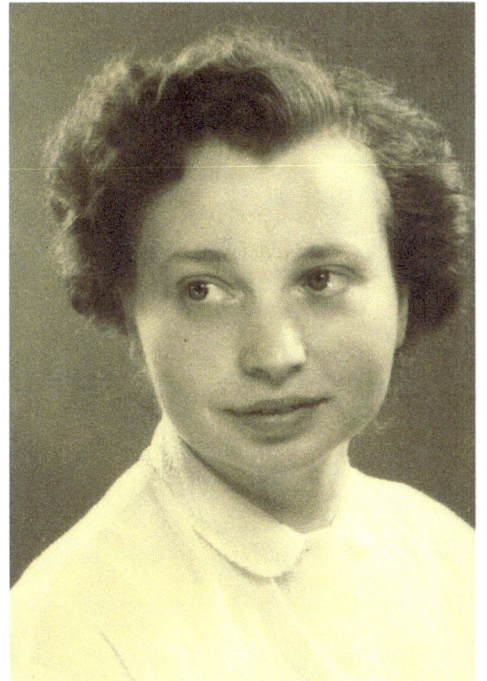

Riet

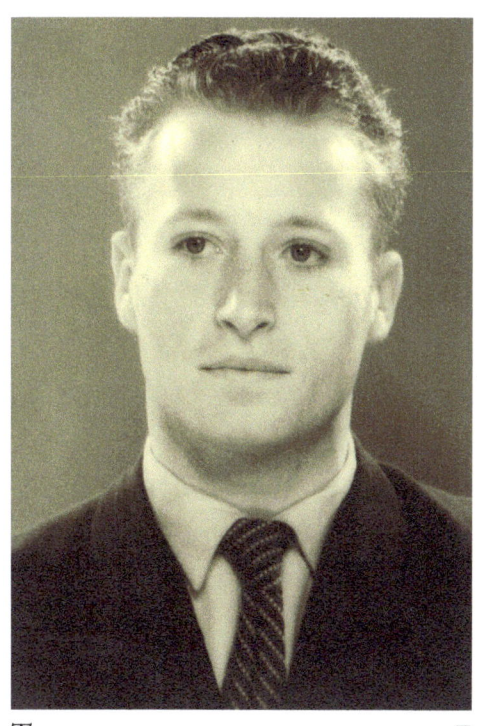

Ton

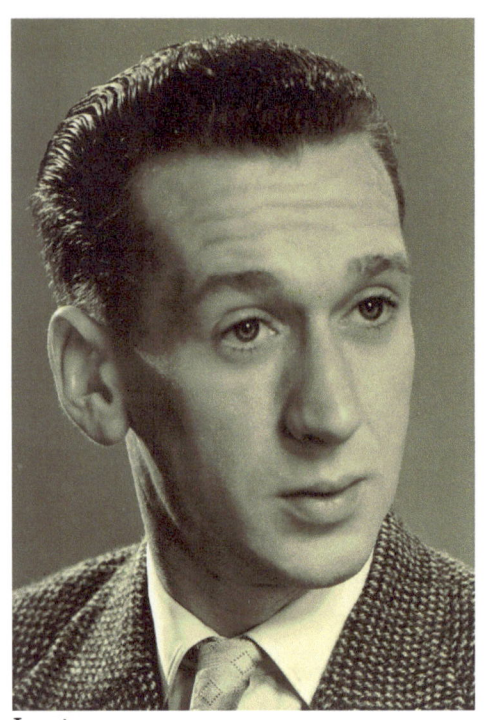
Louis

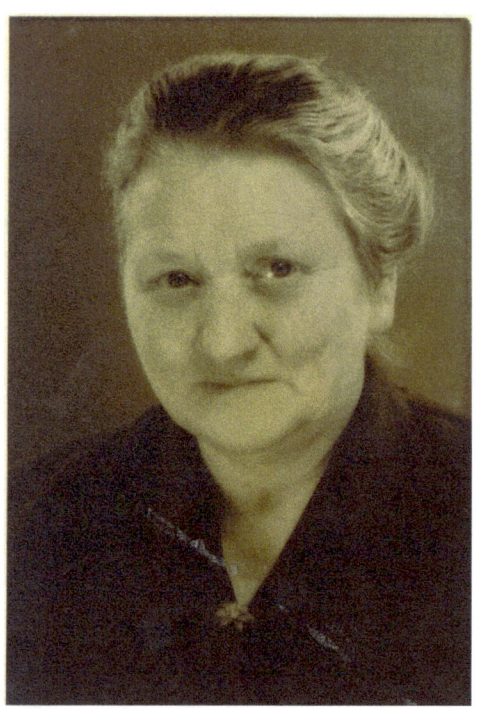
My mother at 68 years

Wedding of Frans and Trus

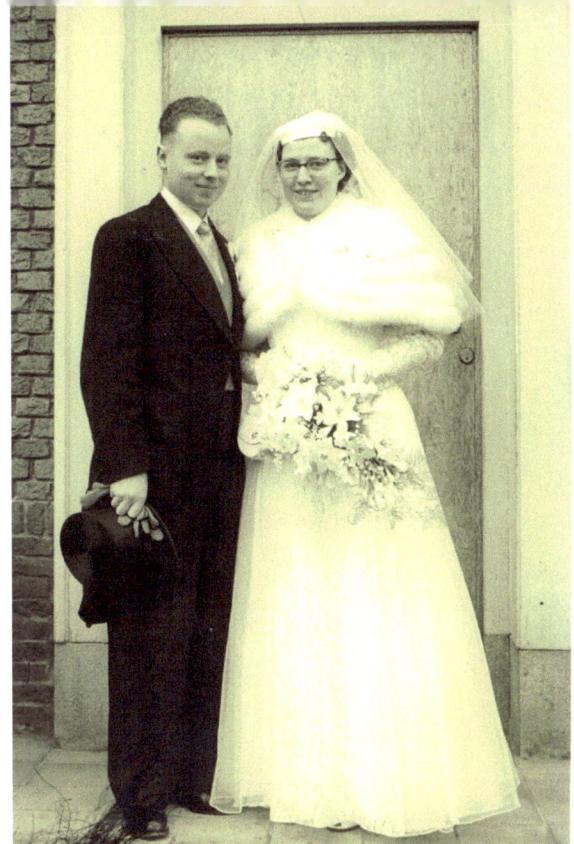

Ben and Kitty's Wedding,
Ans is a bridesmaid

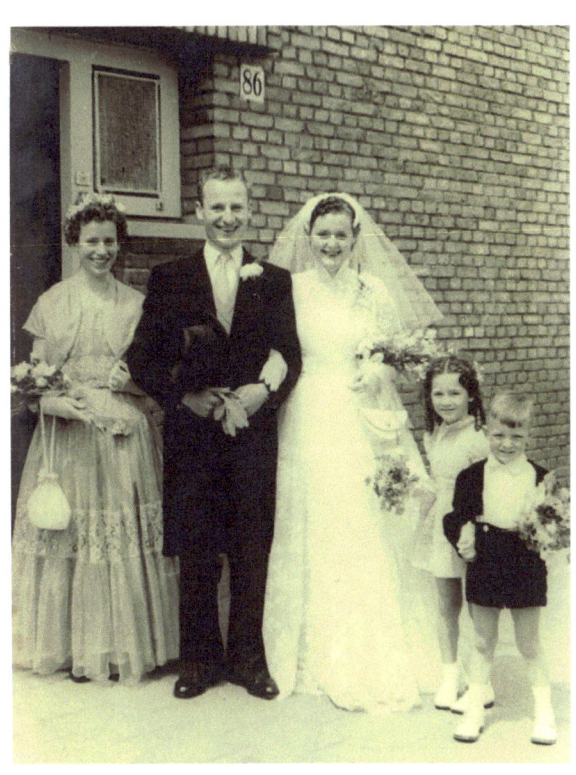

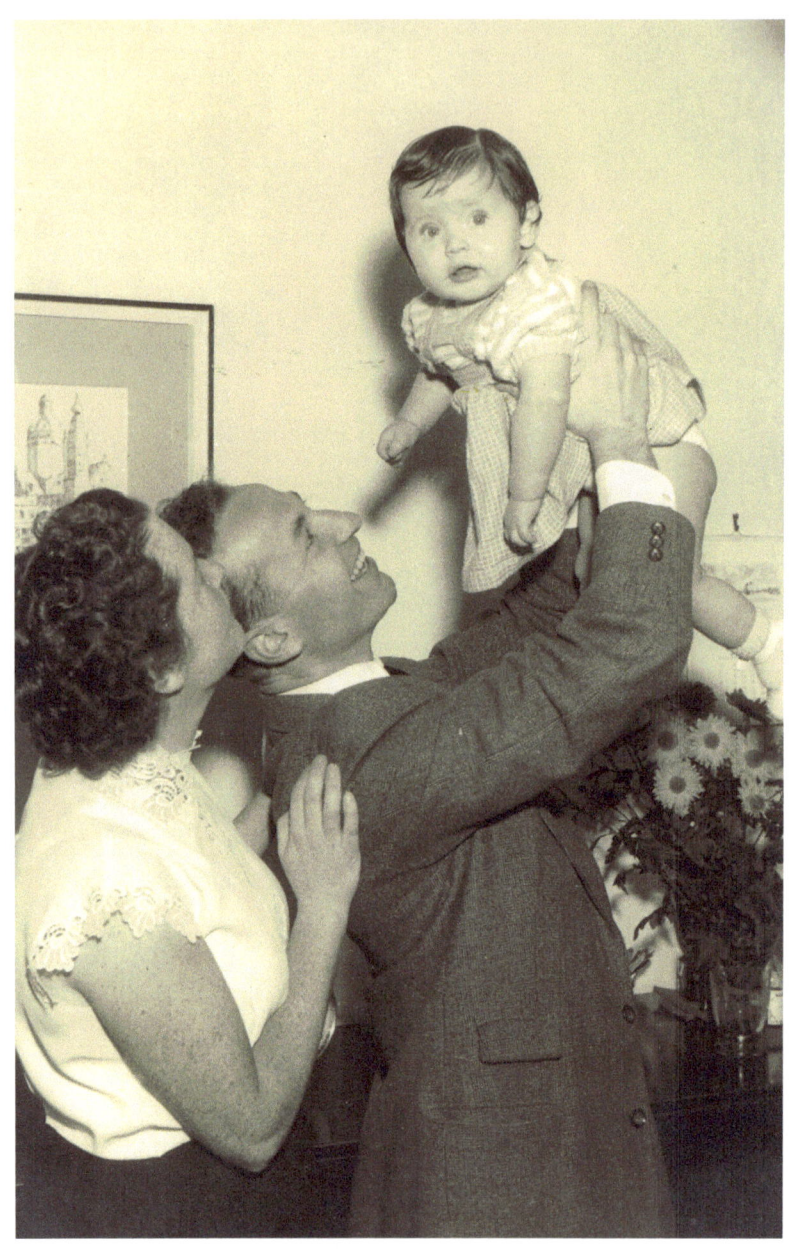

Ben and Kitty with Marja

Our family home on the water is the one at the end

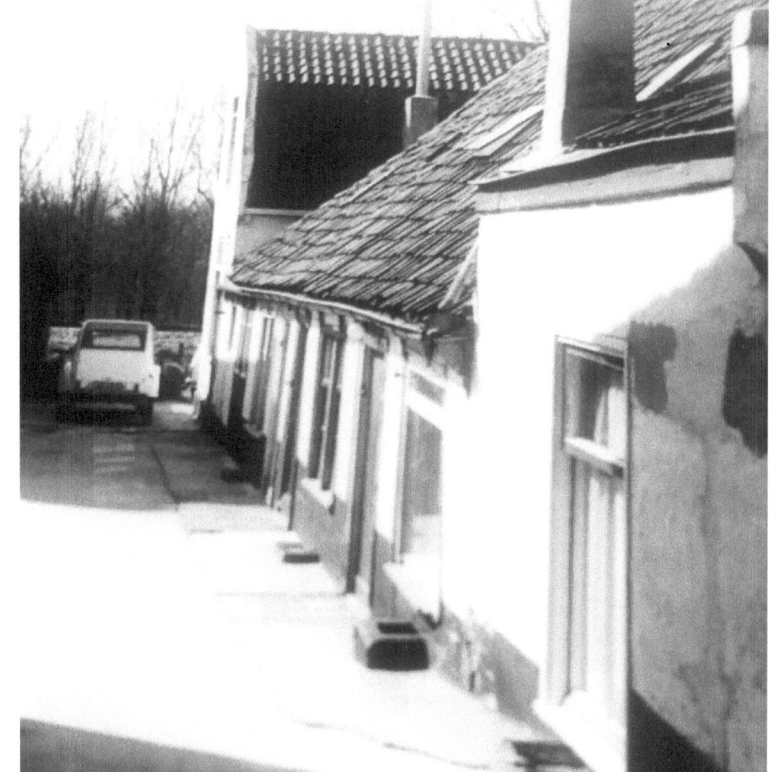

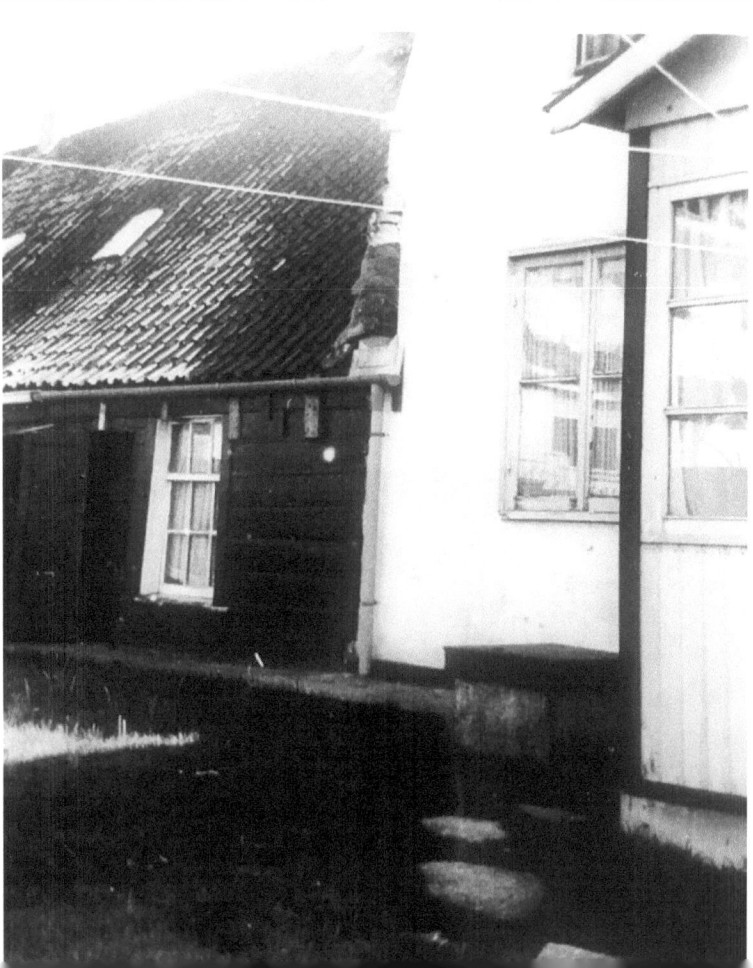

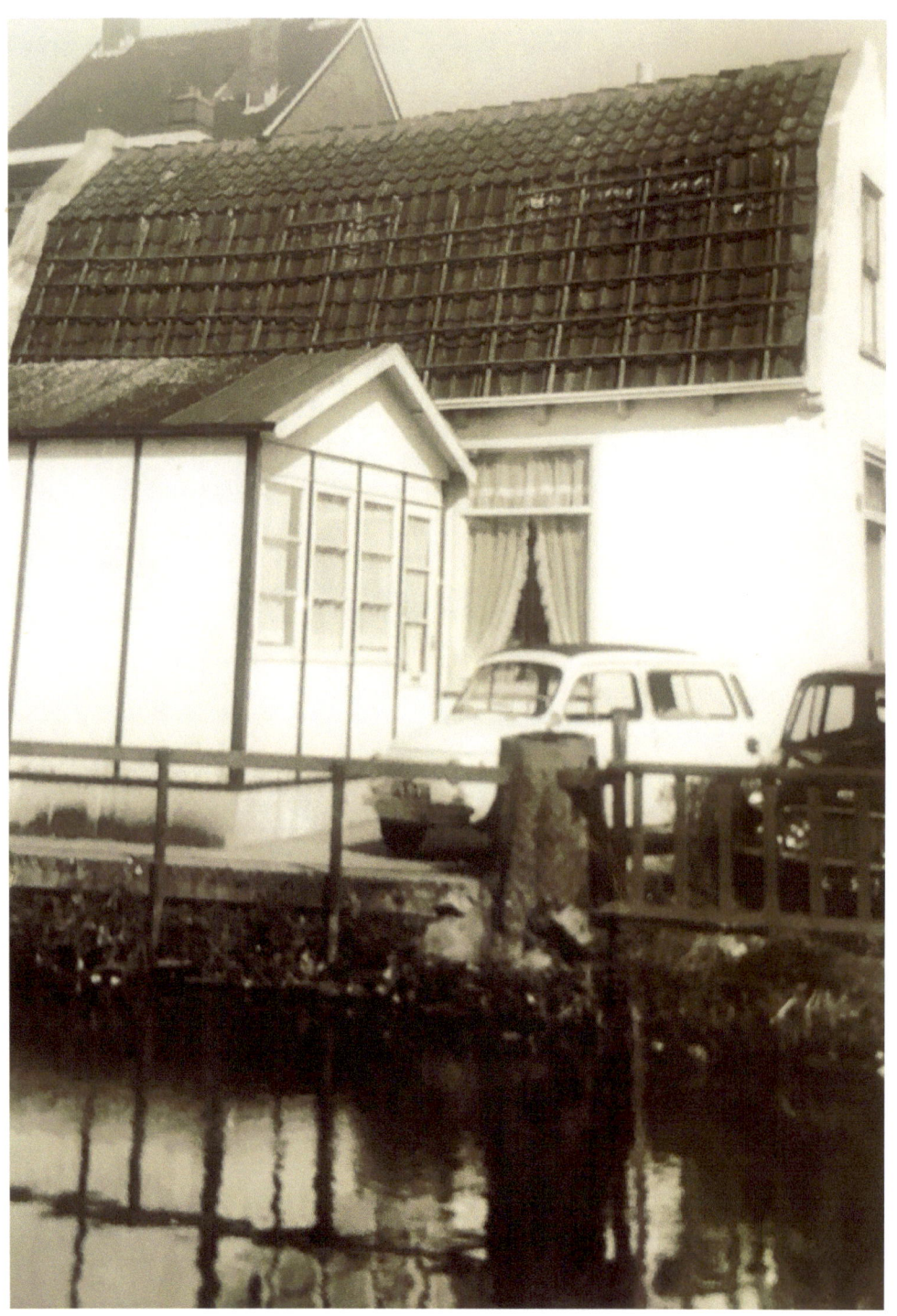

MY TEENAGE YEARS

I started high school in September 1945 and turned thirteen that year. I would ride my bike to school which was a distance of six kilometres. And I had some nice friends, who also rode their bikes. In summer they would sometimes stop at Febo to buy ice cream. I would then ride on home as I did not have any money. My friends often offered to buy me ice cream, but I felt I could never reciprocate, so I did not accept.

The school I went to was a MULO which was a four-year course for students that wanted to become teachers, nurses or clerks to work in offices.

If you wanted to become a tradesman, you went to a trade school for two years after which you did an apprenticeship with a prospective employer. For girls, there was the school of domestic science, where my sister Riet went for two years.

My two eldest brothers went to the trade school. Frans became an electrician and Niek a plumber. Ben, the third one, was considered quite bright by his teachers and did not want to become a tradesman, so he went to the MULO and ended up working at the stock exchange. He became quite successful. He always felt he was a bit better than his brothers and earned the nickname of "The Baron".

The fourth boy, my brother Louis became a carpenter as he was 'no student'. He was always in trouble at school; I remember him often having to write 100 lines for punishment, or sometimes having to draw the map of Germany, which he could do by heart after so many times.

For children of the working class, it was mostly decided by the headmaster what school you would go to after primary school. My parents were wonderful, and they asked us what we wanted to be, and when my dad asked me, and I told him I wanted to be a nurse, he seemed pleased and said, "then you must go to the MULO".

Louis was very talented and could draw well although never having had any art lessons. Art was a subject we all missed out on as during the war, there were no materials, and it was a very low priority in our curriculum, as was music. Louis again loved music and could sing most arias of any opera. I remember on a Sunday afternoon in winter we would all sit in our lounge room reading and listen to the radio. There was always an opera playing on Sundays. This must be where my love of opera stems from.

My younger brother Fons also went to the MULO as did my sister Ans, who became a teacher and my youngest brother Faas, who worked for many years for the equivalent of Telecom. Ton went to the trades school and became a carpenter.

Why I am elaborating on my siblings' education will become clear as during my first year of high achool my father died. He had cancer of the oesophagus, although, at first it was thought that he had a stomach ulcer.

Every night at dinnertime he would take a few bites and say, "I can't eat anymore, I am full!" The doctor treated him for an ulcer, but it did not work. He was admitted to hospital after six weeks and died suddenly while being prepared for surgery.

It was an enormous shock for us all. Not only was my mother left with ten children between the ages of seven and nineteen, but she was left with no income. There was no pension for widows in those days. To make things worse, the child endowment, a payment made to help with bringing up children, was paid on the wages of the breadwinner. When the breadwinner died, the child endowment payments stopped. A shocking anomaly in the law, but that is how it was.

Frans and Niek were both doing an apprenticeship and starting a job, and their wages were the only money coming in. They were giving half their salaries to my mum.

My dad used to work as a gravedigger at the R.C. cemetery. A week after his death the deacon named Boekhorst came to see my mum and handed her an envelope with a week wages saying, "this is the last you will get."

No pension or anything in those days. My mum asked him, "how am I going to feed my children? I am even losing the child endowment payments".

His answer was, "oh, I can help you with that, you can come and sweep and clean the church every morning from 9 'til 12 and I will pay you twenty-five guilders a week. That will then allow you to get the child endowment on your wages."

My mother had no choice but to accept the offer, although she could ill afford to be away from home every morning. She would come home exhausted as sweeping between the benches was hard work. There were services twice a day in those days. Life was very hard for her, but she was tough; I never saw her cry.

I remember her coming home quite upset one day. She said the priest had told her she must clean the tabernacle (a structure above the altar). As this is very high, she asked, "how am I supposed to do that?" He suggested putting a ladder from the choir to the top of the tabernacle and sliding across. Mum refused. The priest insisted it could be done. Mum said, "my children have already lost their father. If I fall, I could be killed. No, I don't want them to lose their mother as well. I won't do it!"

Fortunately, the law that paid the child endowment on the breadwinner's wages was changed, and as soon as my mother was notified of the change, she gave her notice.

The priest was not happy. He said, "if you stop working you will not get the twenty-five guilders a week anymore". My mum answered, "so be it. I have enough work at home, we will have to manage".

The church certainly did not do the right thing by my family.

Some friendly people in our church would now and then put some money in my mother's hand during mass on Sundays. Every bit would help.

My friends had joined the girl guides, and I asked mum if I could join too. She said yes of course, but I cannot afford the weekly contributions, which was twenty-five cents a week.

My brother Niek, who was a scout said he would give me twenty-five cents a week to keep all his shoes polished. He had a pair of work boots, which I had to polish every day. Plus one pair he wore after work when he went out, and a pair he only wore on Sundays. I just needed to polish his Sunday shoes on Monday. If I ever forgot to polish one of his shoes, he would not pay me for that week, and still expected me to keep polishing that week. I thought that was very mean! I was usually very good at the job. I wonder now how my mother allowed him to be so cruel. I suppose it taught me not to slacken off.

I loved the girl guide meetings and come summer we were to go on a camp! I had never been on any holiday yet and very much wanted to go. But it cost fifteen guilders, which my mum did not have.

I had heard about a farmer looking for kids to pick beans, so I went to see him and was taken on for three weeks picking at five guilders a week. Perfect! Now I could go on the camp!

We had a lot of fun, and I loved the camp. We had a kind leader named Truus Peters. She decided that as none of us could swim that she would take us to an indoor pool for the next term instead of our regular meetings in the clubhouse.

I was quite terrified as we had to jump into the deep end and the attendant would hook an iron loop around our head and drag you along. What a strange way to teach you how to swim, but I somehow passed the exam at the end as did all the other girls. We only learned breaststroke and backstroke, but I was ever so grateful to our leader as in those days there was no school swimming, and some of my siblings never learned to swim.

I enjoyed high school and was good at languages and most subjects, except history.

I think that was mainly due to my best friend Betsy Nordsiek, who used to say: why do we have to learn about all these dead people? Being a teenager,

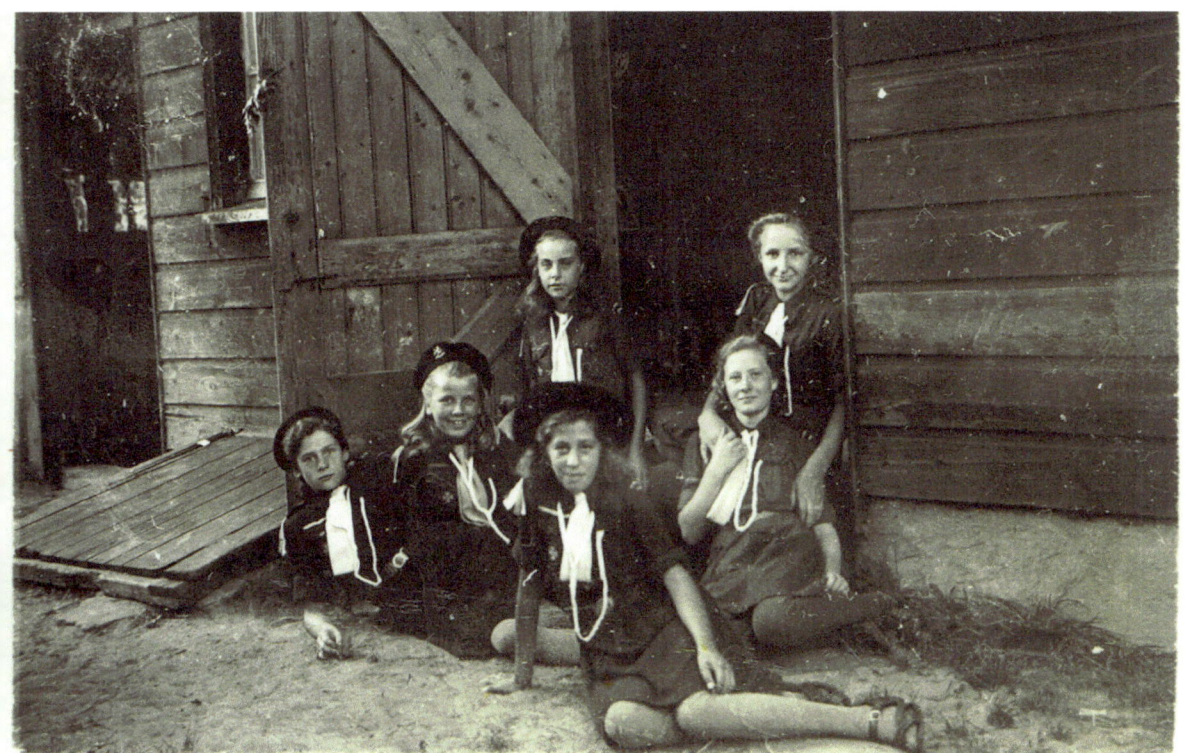

Girl guide camp

when your best friend hates something, it seems that you hate it too.

I remember when our exams were close the history teacher gave some extra lessons. I was excluded. She said to me, "you have never shown any interest. You don't come to the extra lessons". Okay, I thought, I did not care.

Our exams were always oral in those days

When my turn came I was sitting in front of three examiners. The first question they asked me was, "do you like history?" I paused for a while and said, "that is a tough question!" They asked, "Why?" I answered, "because you all obviously do and I have to be honest and say that, no, I don't like history".

They seemed surprised at my answer and started by asking me some elementary questions. When I knew the answer, I would elaborate, and when I did not know the answer, I would say so. As there was a time limit, I would drag my answers out at least what I knew.

When time was up, they said, "well, for someone who does not like history you did not do too badly".

The next day the history teacher read out the exam results. When she came to my name and read eighty percent, she was furious. "How could you get eighty percent? You know nothing!" I was not really a particularly clever child, but I was crafty!

I was now sixteen years old and had finished my education necessary for nursing, but I was too young. One had to be nineteen, so what to do next? Some of my friends found jobs in offices, but I did not like the idea of working in an office. As I had been babysitting for a family lately on occasion, the lady asked me if I wanted to work for her. Helping with housework and looking after the children. We did not talk about a wage, and as a babysitter, I had been paid quite well, so I left it up to them. When I got my first pay-packet, I was very disappointed. I got far less than I had been getting as a babysitter. But still, I was working very hard and enjoyed the children.

Once the seventh baby was born, the lady liked to go out on a Saturday afternoon with her husband. I was left in charge of the children and some chores. It is funny how you remember some things, but one Saturday the parents came home, and I got told off because there was a small potato peel next to the bin instead of in it! I had been rushing to get all the chores done. Peel the veggies for the evening meal and keep the children happy. I felt very hurt!

As I had been talking to my friends about what they were earning, which was much more than what I was getting, I decided to look for an office job and quit my job as a home help. Though, it had not at all been a waste of six months, as I learned a lot and years later I was glad of the experience when I worked as a maternity nurse in the community.

My office job was simple. It was in the centre of Amsterdam in the Kalverstraat. Anyone familiar with Amsterdam will know that the Kalverstraat runs between the Dam Plein and the Munt Plein. The work was easy! Some typing and a lot of filing. Our office was on the third floor, and the rest of the business was on the first floor. When there was no work to be done, we would read a book. I enjoyed my lunchtime walks in the city, and as I was earning more, I could contribute a bit more at home and save up for my nursing outfit.

My mother was always very fair. She used to say that, "you can all become whatever you want." We all used to give mum half of our wages which covered most expenses and as the family grew things became more comfortable. We all reached our potential more or less.

I never contributed much as once I started my nursing training most of my pay went into board and lodging as we used to live in the nurses home attached to the hospital. My teenage years were happy years. I joined a theatrical group and enjoyed acting. Many years later I met up with one of the group quite by chance in Johannesburg at the airport. We became good friends.

I also became a cub leader. Having enjoyed my years as a girl guide, I was happy to oblige when I was asked to become a cub leader. There were three leaders in our troupe, and we became good friends.

In the summer holidays, we took the cubs on a camp which everyone enjoyed very much.

Me at 18 as a cub leader

BECOMING & BEING A NURSE

Once I turned nineteen, I applied to the RKZ (Roman Catholic Hospital) in Hilversum to start my nursing training. I started in February 1953.

There was a new course beginning every six months. There were eleven students in our group between the ages of nineteen and twenty-one. The hospital had 120 beds and was run by nuns. Male and female wards were separated. There was a male surgical ward and a female surgical ward, and the same for the medical wards. Each department had a large ward with twenty beds and a smaller ward with ten beds. And two private rooms for the very seriously ill patients. There was also a children's ward and a special ward for private patients, who would have their own room. Then there was a maternity wing with a labour ward, and of course an operating theatre.

As student nurses, we would spend three months at least in each ward during our three-year training, except the maternity ward as that was an additional six-month training after general nursing. We were lucky if we got time in the operating theatre and fortunate if we got to scrub up for a minor operation such as an appendectomy. We all found that a most exciting time.

There was only one bathroom to each ward with a bath, no shower.

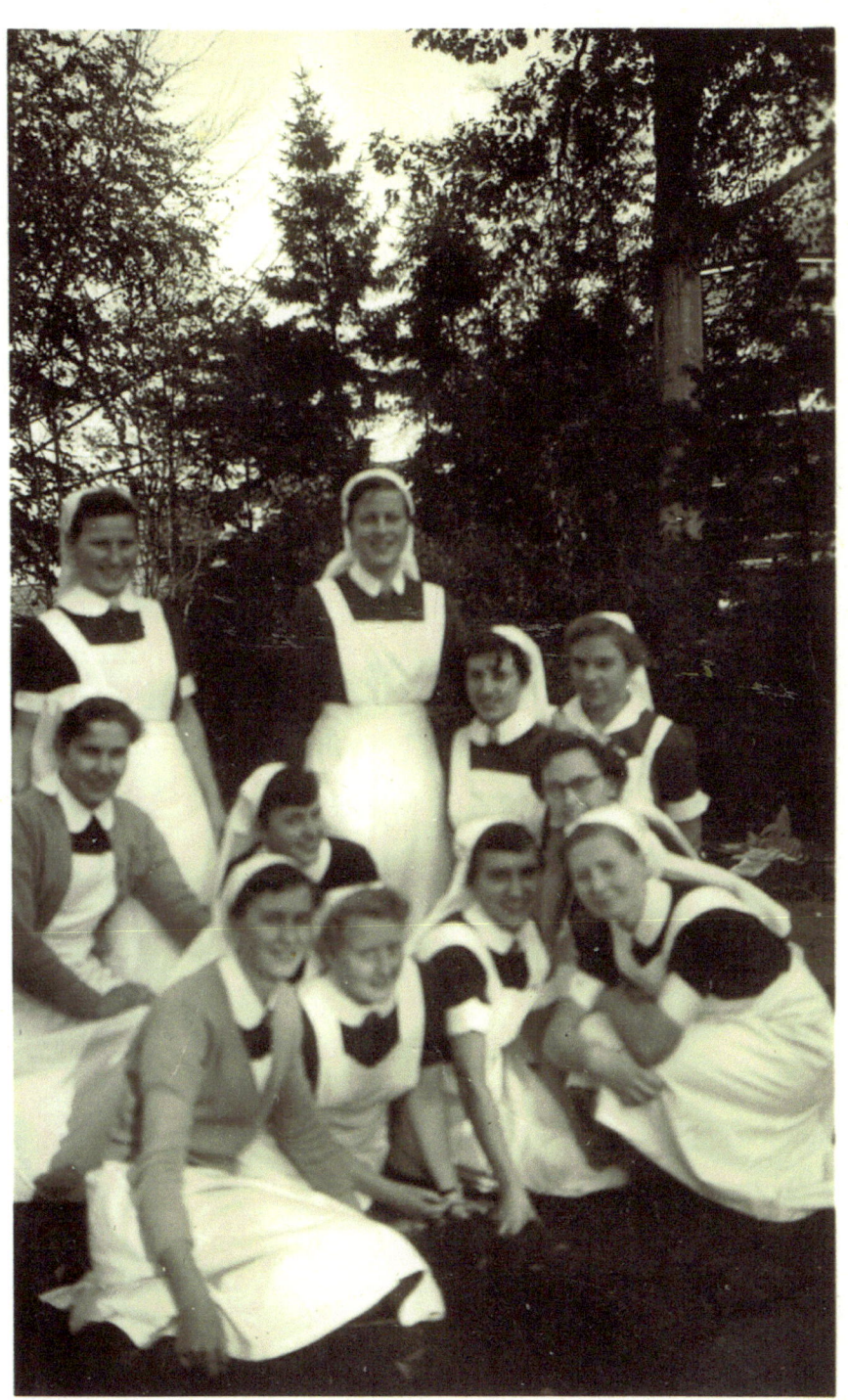
My year of eleven trainee nurses

Patients seldom got to use it. Personal hygiene was very different in those days. Everyone was nursed in bed. The men had urinals and had to use a bedpan for number two. The women always had to use a bedpan.

The night staff used to pass a bowl to each patient to wash their face and hands in the early morning. When on night duty you were not allowed to start passing bowls and bedpans until 5 am. Then you would collect and empty all the urinals and bedpans. Then, you had to quickly tidy the beds and give any insulin injections if there were any diabetic patients in your care. Everything had to be finished at 7 am because the priest would come with communion. If your ward was not tidy, you would be in trouble. Can you imagine? Thirty-two patients on your own to do all that in two hours! No wonder I used to hate night duty!

We were thrown in at the deep end. In the first six months we had to learn so much!

How to give a bed bath and how to wash a patient's bottom as that was the first thing the day staff would do. Everyone had their bottom washed! Nurses today would have a good laugh thinking about that, but that is what the routine was. Then we had to learn how to make a bed with or without a patient in it and how to clean a bed after a patient went home. Remember there were no orderlies to do those things.

We had to learn how to collect urine and faeces and sputum for the lab. The only specimens we did not collect was blood. We also did the cleaning of the wards and of the bedpans and urinals and sputum pots, which was a foul job, but we all had to take turns. It seems ridiculous now, but we even cut up a piece of fruit for each patient and looked after their flowers.

Before anaesthetic machines were used, patients were anaesthetised with chloroform and ether, and almost everyone was sick afterwards. So we did a lot of cleaning up of kidney dishes, if they managed to use those, or worse if they didn't.

Nurses these days think they work hard, and yes they do, but in many ways, the work has become a lot easier. We even had to rinse all the dirty laundry before it went to the laundry!

A typical day would start with a mass at 7 am, followed by a quick breakfast of bread and jam or cheese or cold meat and a cup of tea, and you had to be on the ward by 7:45 am. The sister in charge would read the report and delegate the morning's work. We would serve morning tea after all the bottoms were washed and the beds were made.

The young student nurses would then get on with their particular job for a week. This could be flower and fruit duty or 'slob sink' (the laundry where it all happened) or washing all bedside lockers and the floors! Yes, we did that too! We would work until 1 pm and then have lunch and a break until 4 pm. Then we would work again until 7 pm. We only had one day off a week and only a weekend after night duty.

We were housed in the nurse's quarters attached to the hospital. Two students to a room, and shared bathrooms with showers.

Meals were simple for patients as well as for nurses. Bread with cheese or cold meat and tea for breakfast. A cooked lunch of meat and veggies, fish on Fridays, and sandwiches at night with sometimes soup. As we were serving the meals the patients always got fed if they could not manage themselves. Not like I have noticed many times today: if a patient is asleep or not able to feed themselves the kitchen staff just takes the tray away without telling the nurses that this patient has not eaten.

We had to learn to give injections before we went on night duty and we used to go on night duty after six months. We knew very little and had the responsibility of caring for thirty-two patients. When in doubt we could call on a third year roving nurse, and she would check on us a few times during the night. She would be the one to call a doctor if needed.

The first few times, we were terrified to be alone at night. Fortunately, we only did a week at the time. Usually one week out of six and then we got a weekend off, which we all enjoyed.

I always went home for my days off and travelled mostly by train, but sometimes I had no money left for the train, and then I rode my bike. It was thirty kilometres, and it took me two hours. I did not mind not having much money but felt bad that I could not contribute at home where things were still tight. The two youngest siblings were still studying, but none of my siblings ever made an adverse remark. I always had stories to tell, and they all seemed to

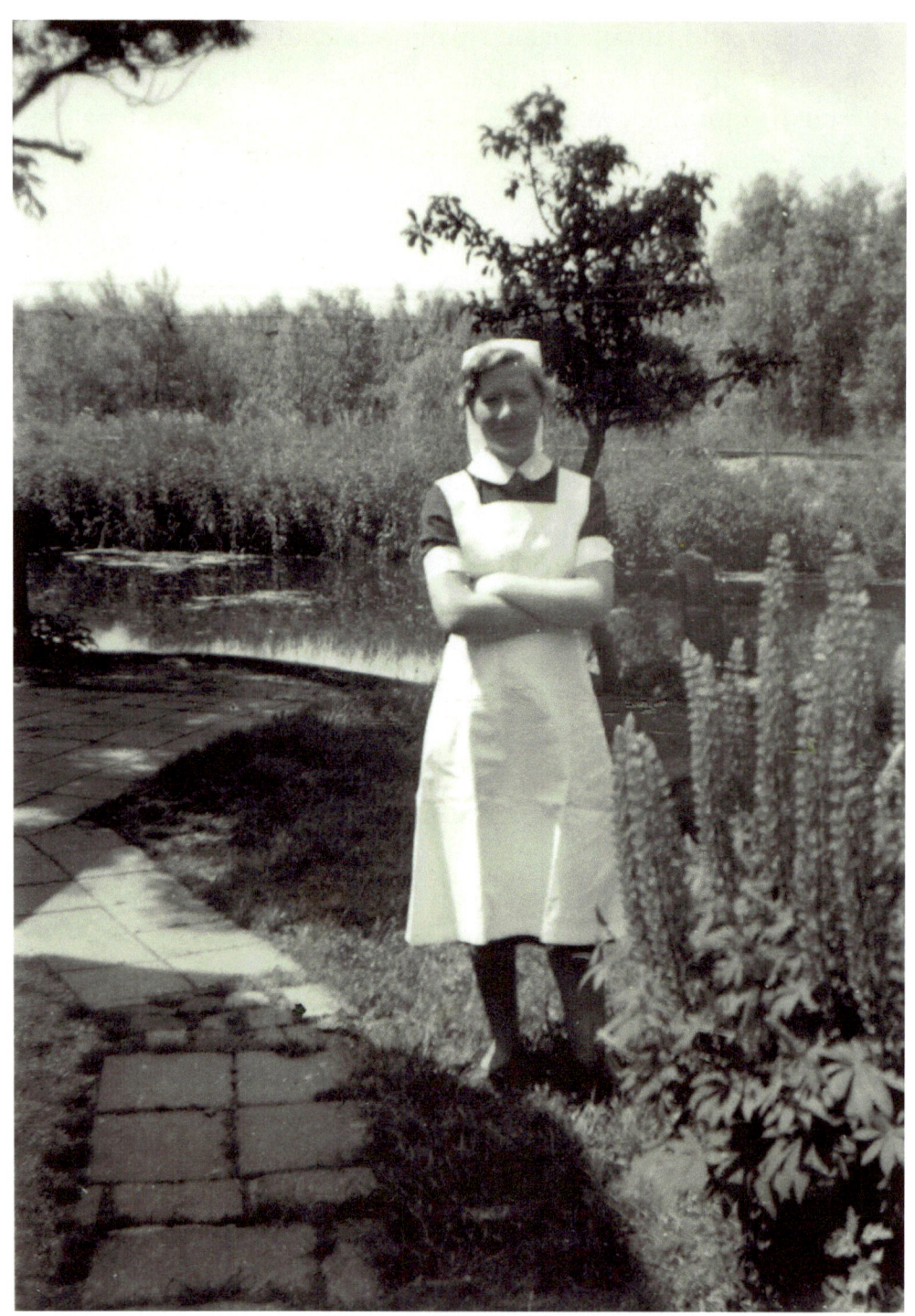

At home in the garden

enjoy me coming home as much as I did.

I made some very good friends during my three years in Hilversum. My best friend was, and still is, Els Schweitzer. She lived in Bussum, which is close to Hilversum, so she went home more often. I sometimes went with her.

I remember how her dear mother was very gullible. We used to tease her and tell her the most ridiculous stories, and she believed us. Until we burst out laughing and she would say, "oh, you again."

I also remember how the third-year nurses used to play tricks on us. When someone died, we had to take the body to the mortuary. We did not like that,

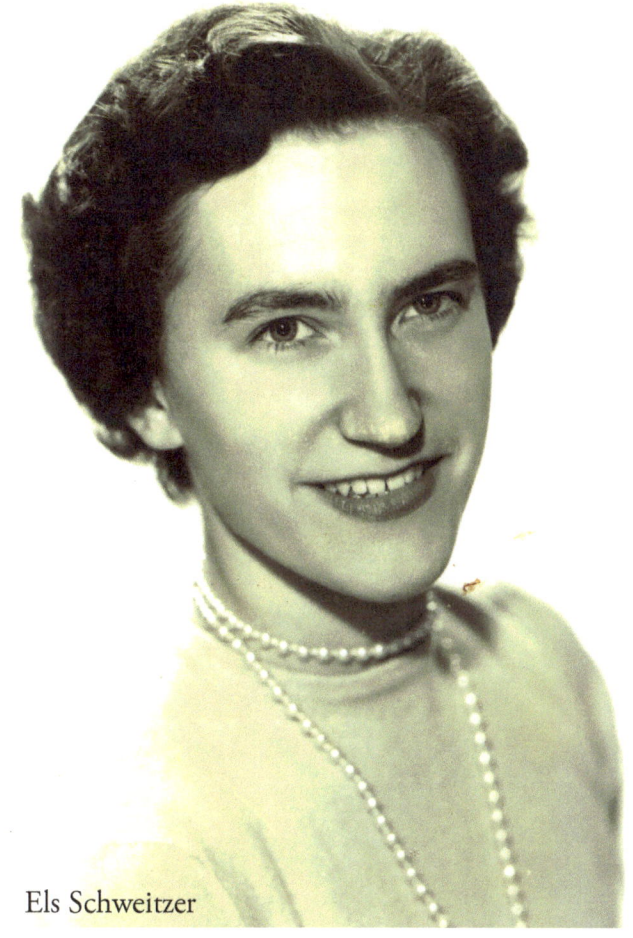

Els Schweitzer

especially at night. One night, while lifting the body on an empty slab, nurse Schillings, a third-year student, had hidden under a sheet on the next slab and slowly got up, making a dreadful noise. I nearly died I got such a fright. One reason I still remember her name today, Marian Schillings.

Tuesday was lecture day. We left the ward for an hour at a time, and one very sweet nun Sister Josefia would teach us nursing care. Most specialists working at the hospital were involved with training us. We were like one big family. One surgeon, Dr Schmedding, would teach us chirurgy and Dr Sandberg, an internist, would teach us internal medicine. The ENT specialist would teach us all about ear, nose and throat diseases. It was an excellent system. We could often relate the condition to a patient we were nursing.

The biggest plus was that we could support ourselves on a very small wage. Nurses earned very little but with board and lodging provided one could manage. Today with university training it is much harder if you have no support from home.

In our third year, we were all making plans where to do our maternity training. This was a six-month course where you learned to assist the doctor with a birth, either in a hospital or at home as there were many home births then. My mother had all her eleven children at home. (One died at two weeks old). Because she had a nurse taking care of her and the baby and all the other children, she used to say that was her annual holiday.

I wanted to do my maternity training in Amsterdam while living at home, and so did my friend Ria Kuyer. Alas, Ria failed her final exam and had to repeat six months, so I went on my own. I rode my bike to the hospital every day, which was about twelve kilometres. The hospital was the OLVG (Our Dear Lady Hospital.) I enjoyed my six months there.

I kept in touch with my friends in Hilversum during that time, especially my friend Jackie Vocking, as she had similar aspirations as I had, namely working in an underdeveloped country. Jackie was in a group that finished six months after me, so she finished her general when I finished my maternity training. I decided to wait for her so that we might go somewhere together.

My brother Ben and his wife Kitty had their first baby Marja, while I was working in Amsterdam. Marja could not wait until she was at the hospital and was almost born in a taxi. I was present at the birth and got to look after them while in hospital.

Mother and baby used to stay in the hospital for ten days. We used to weigh the baby before and after each feed, and if the baby had not had enough, we used to complement with a bottle. No demand feeding then, and it was custom to feed every three hours. How things have changed! No disposable nappies and all the bottles had to be boiled to sterilise.

Washing nappies was a daily chore taking up a lot of time and energy for the mother, but then, they did not go out much while the baby was small. Today's mums are so busy with all the activities the children taking part in, which is probably just as tiring as washing the nappies, and certainly more expensive.

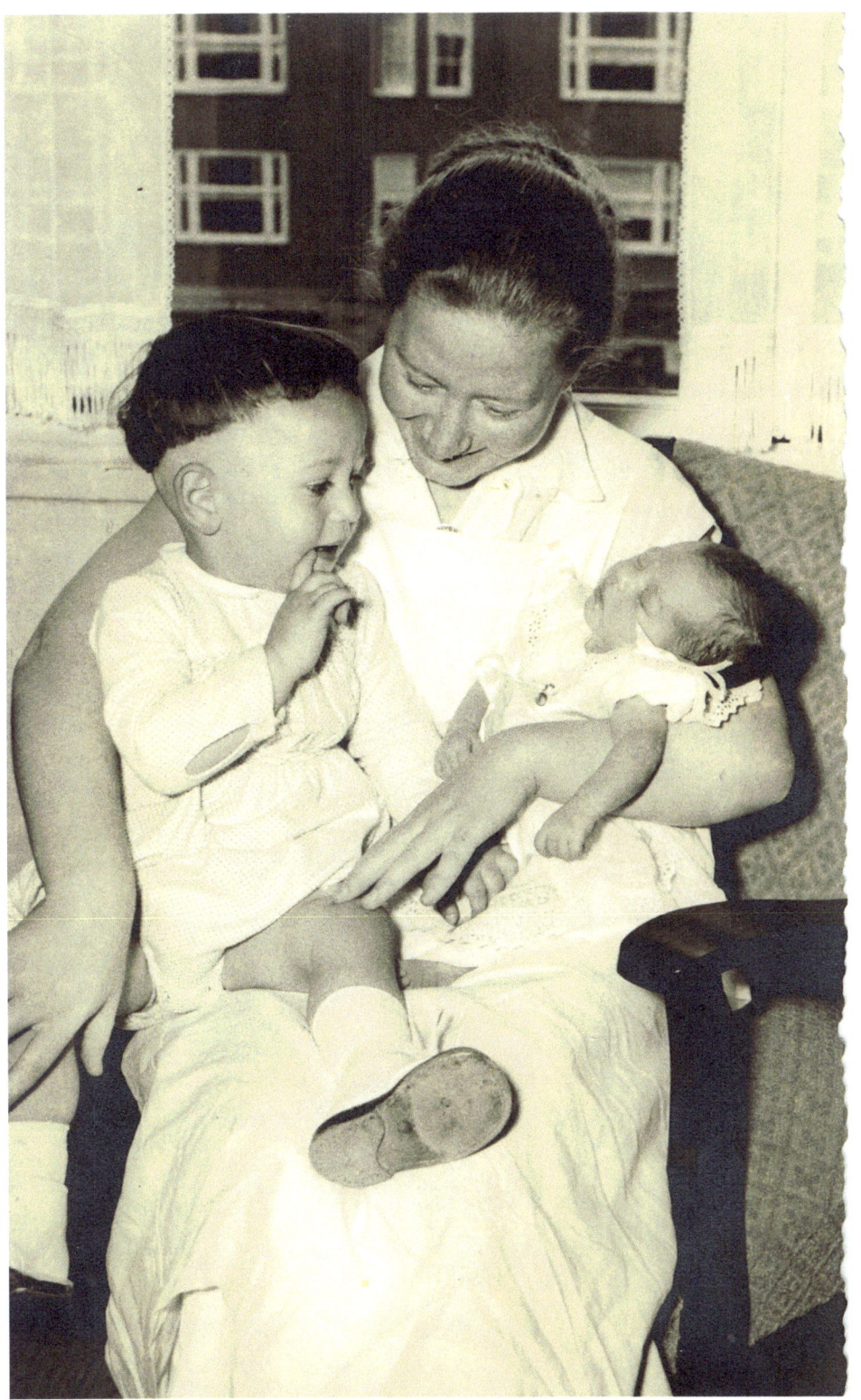

1957, Maternity nursing in the district

I did some private nursing during the next six months while waiting for Jackie. We had decided to go to New Guinea together.

When you were a private maternity nurse, you took over the care of mother and baby during confinement and also look after any other children plus the cooking and housekeeping. My niece was expecting her seventh baby and asked me if I would do her confinement. I agreed, and that was the most difficult one of all my cases.

I had to have a smallpox vaccination for New Guinea as I was never immunised as a child against smallpox. My niece happened to go into labour the day after I had my vaccination. I felt I could not let her down, so I went and worked really hard with that family, but boy was I sick! I was running a high temp, and should not have continued, but fortunately, all worked out. In hindsight, I should not have done it.

Jackie and I had both been accepted and first had to do a six-week course in tropical diseases and emergency medicine. We both very much wanted to go to an outpost. We had to do some tests, and one test was to draw a tree! I had a good think about that and thought: What are they looking for? A person who is stable and well-grounded? So, I drew a tree that had as many roots underground as branches above ground.

When we got our appointments, Jackie was placed in Merauke a small city on the South Coast with a good size hospital. I got posted in the centre of NG (New Guinea) to a tiny settlement with one doctor and two nurses, me and one Indonesian-trained nurse. I was delighted, and Jackie was very disappointed. Why did I get the placement? I wondered, was it the tree? I will never know.

The Dutch government was putting a lot of effort in the last colony after they lost Indonesia and sent many teachers, doctors and nurses to even very remote places. The Eastern part of NG was under Australian rule, but the Dutch had always neglected the Western half. Indonesia did not want it, so it was still under Dutch control.

Apart from the various Missions, not much had been done, but this was changing now. Over the years Indonesia had sent teachers to many outposts with the result that some of the Papuas had learned a bit of the language, which came in very handy as there were so many different local languages, making it impossible to communicate. Each village seemed to have their own language.

During our six-week course, we learned a few basics, and I bought a good dictionary which proved a great help.

Of the tropical diseases, we learned malaria was number one. It was easy to diagnose by taking a drop of blood and putting it under the microscope, but I soon learned that if a patient presented with a fever and has a headache, it is usually malaria, so we would treat the patient with quinine. All personnel were advised to take 'Paludrine' prophylactically, and that was very effective as I never got malaria in the three and a half years I was there. I did, however, get amoebic dysentery after three months, but I recovered after medication and bed rest for a week.

Infant mortality was very high in New Guinea. Partly due to the poor nutrition of the mothers. Breastmilk often had poor nutritional value due to a poor diet, and then some tribes had strange beliefs. For example, that the first breastmilk (colostrum) was poisonous to the baby and therefore was expressed and wasted. Of course, the baby would starve for the first two days and had a very poor start in life.

As it is a vast country with no infrastructure, no roads and very few towns with hospitals, we still knew very little about the population. We had so much to learn, but we were eager to do our best, and the Dutch Government was willing to provide lots of resources and sent many people and provisions. After all, it was the only colony left after Indonesian Independence.

I was to leave in February 1958. It was winter in Holland, so it was impossible to buy enough summer clothes. I had six dresses made and bought jungle boots, sandals, uniforms and I also was to provide my own furniture. I would have two rooms in the hospital. A bedroom and a lounge room.

My luggage left before me by ship, and I would fly later.

I remember the day before I left I cried all day. I was already so homesick! It suddenly dawned on me that I was leaving home for three long years.

My dear mother said to me, "you know, you don't *have* to go! I answered, "I know, but I want to go, but I will miss you all so much!" Remember, in those days there was no telephone, and letters would take weeks to arrive.

The whole family brought me to the airport.

I was flying in a DC9, and the flight to Biak took thirty-six hours with one fuel stop in Karachi. In Biak, I had to wait for a connecting flight to Tanah

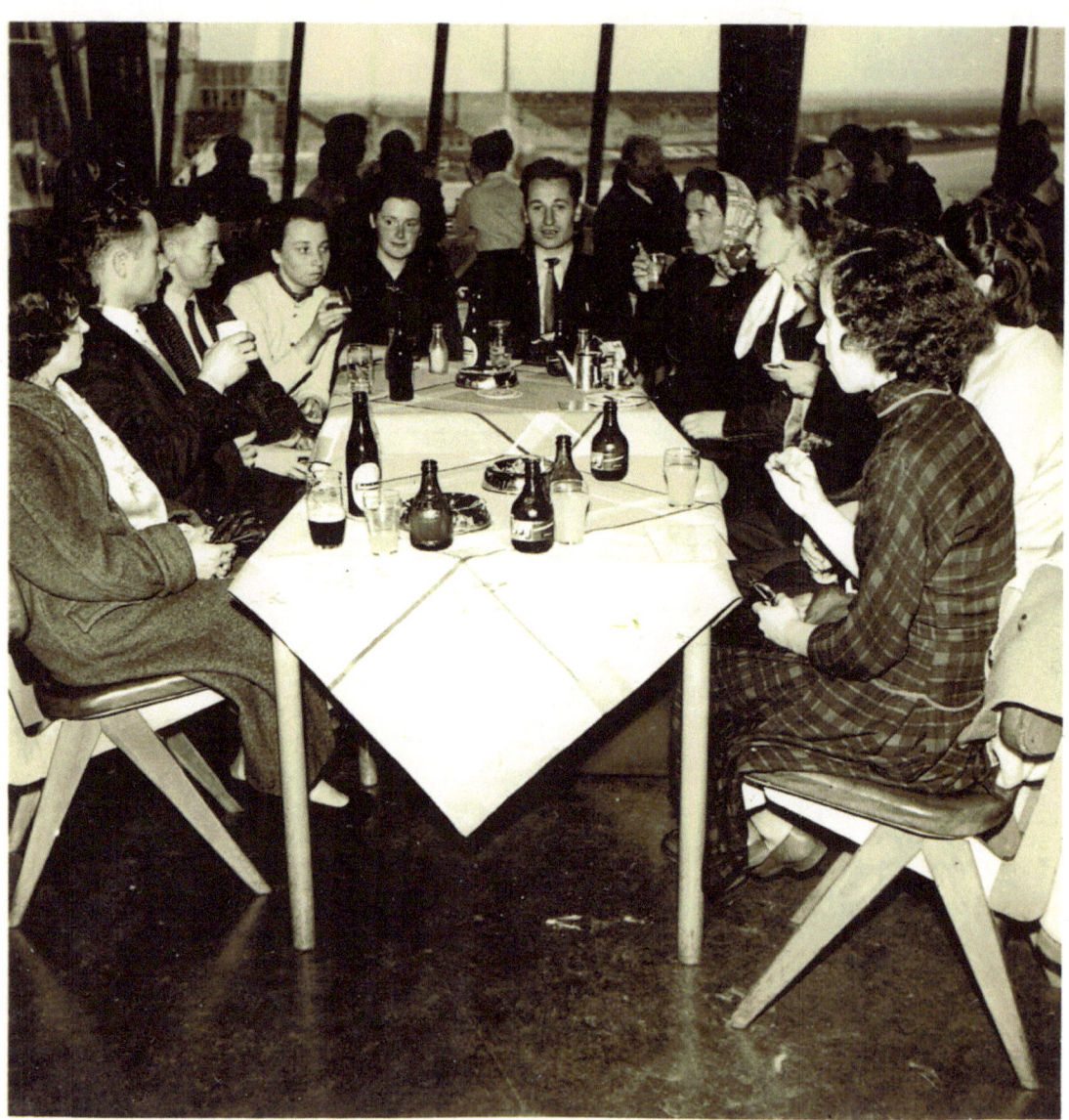

Feb 1958, Last drink before flying to New Ginea

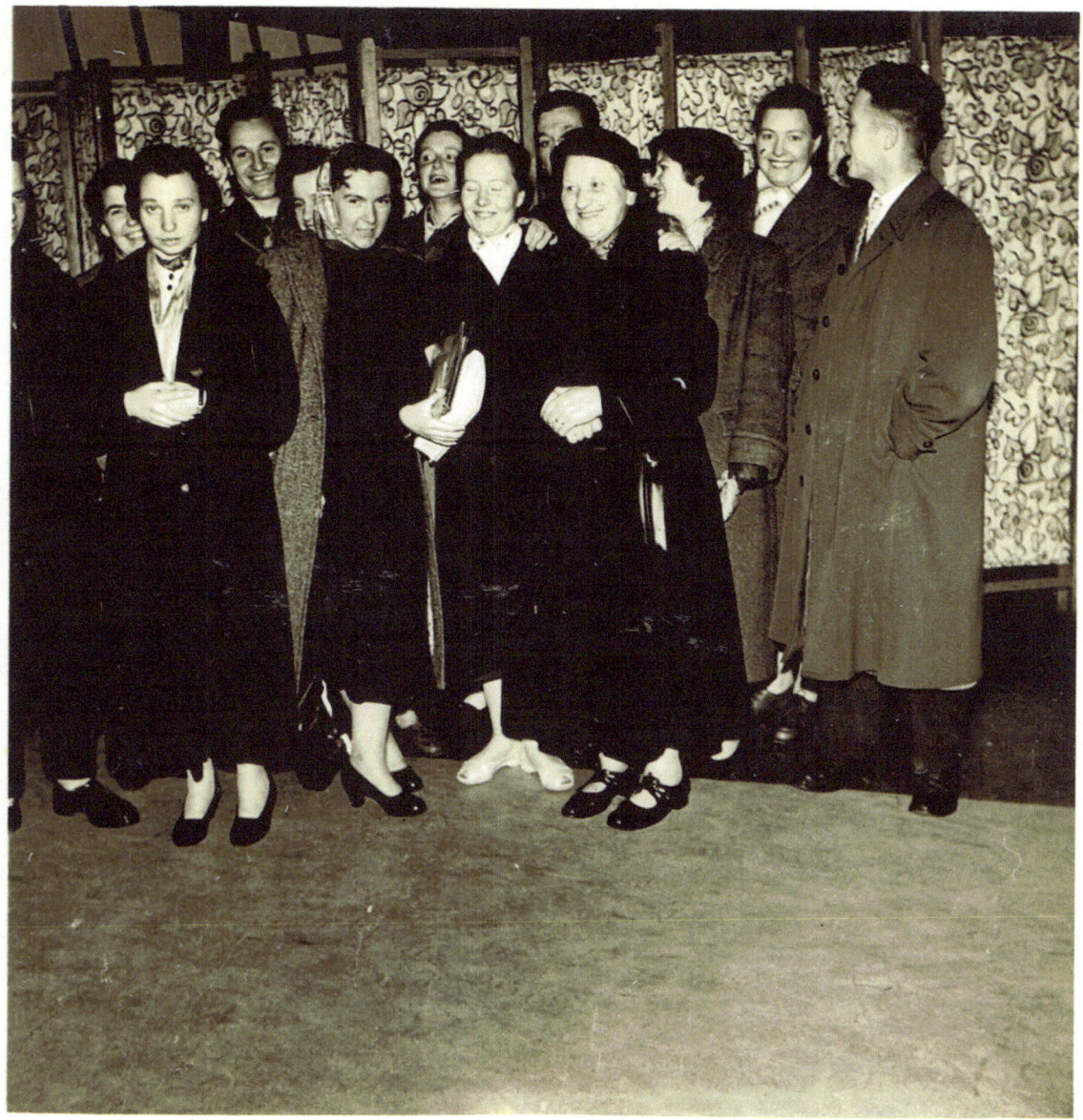
Feb 1958, Schipol airport, the whole family came to see me off to New Ginea

Merah, my ultimate destination.

I remember being so hot! From a freezing Holland to forty degrees celcius in Biak was terrible. I changed and showered at the airport, but I still could not stand it. So, I would keep going to have showers until someone asked me, "where are you off to all the time?" I said, "I am so hot, I have to shower". He told me just to relax and sit down. "You will get used to it".

I was thinking, "What have I done? I will never get used to this".

But of course, I did, although it took a few weeks. There was no air conditioning or even fans in those days. We only had a small fridge for some medications, so no cold drinks or the likes. But then we did not have a refrigerator at home either, so I did not miss that. And as Tanah Merah is inland, there was never a sea breeze either.

TANAH MERAH

When the small plane landed, the whole village had come out to welcome me. Or was it to see what the new nurse looked like? Tanah Merah (meaning 'red earth') was a small settlement in the middle of the jungle. It was there because of the prison.

Headhunting was still a very practised custom amongst the Papuas. But as it had been declared illegal by the Dutch government, perpetrators were caught and put in prison.

It was an open prison, as prisoners would not try to escape. They were mostly so far away from their homeland that they would never make it home with all different tribes around, who might be after their head. People in town could hire a prisoner to work in their garden. The prison had a large vegetable garden where they grew their own food.

The hospital employed two prisoners. One to do the washing, all by hand of course; his name was Kametik. And another named Willibrordus was employed as the cook. When their tribal name was too difficult to pronounce they were given another name while in prison.

The head of the local government was called the HPB which was in my

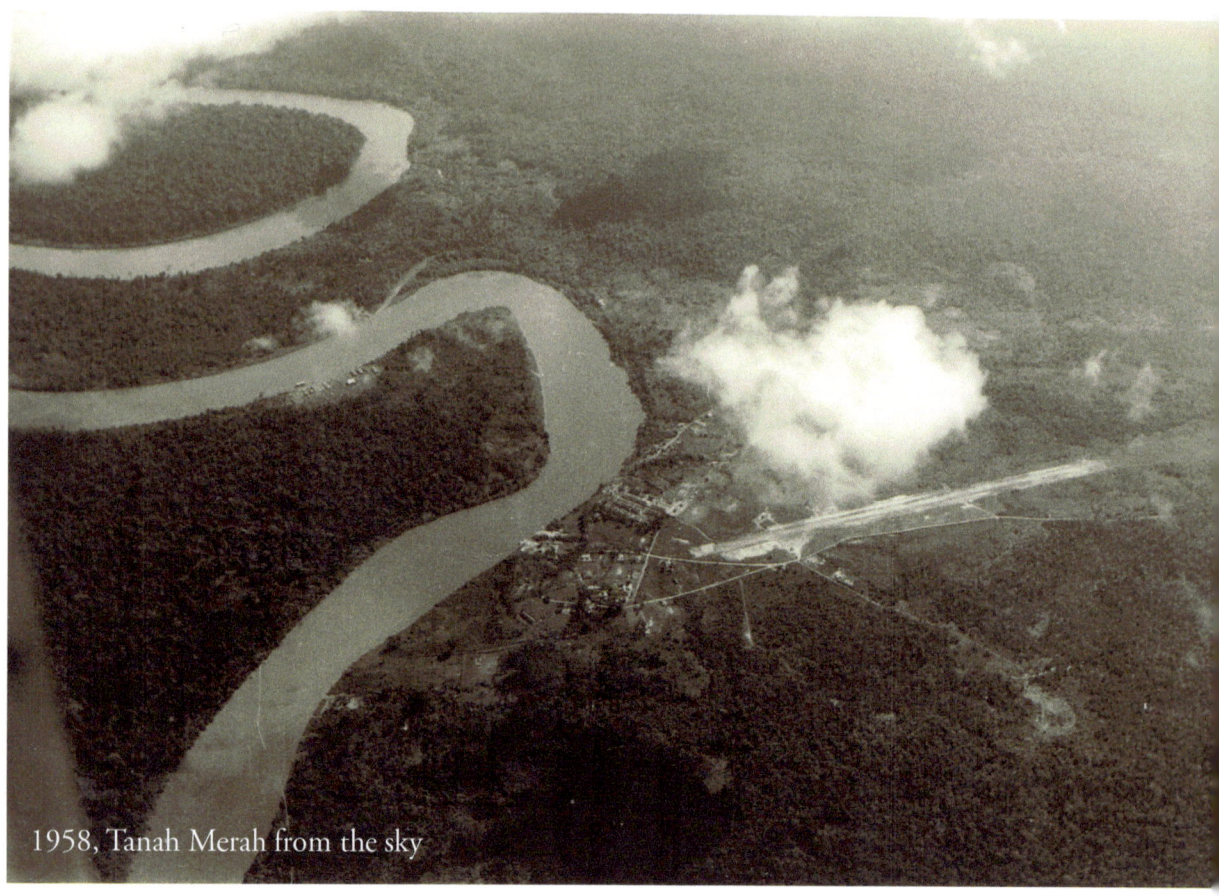
1958, Tanah Merah from the sky

time Frans Peters; he was married to Sonja, and they had a baby girl called Ciska.

Then there was the Dr Henk and his wife Loes Bijkerk and their baby son Ruud.

Henk was not only running the small hospital and daily clinic but had to do surveys of a large district, which took him away from home every second month. Travel was usually by foot as there were no roads. There was a river running through Tanah Merah (The Digul River) so sometimes they could use a prahu part of the way.

We had one Indonesian trained nurse called Leo and a locally trained nurse called Makamur. One of them would go with Henk on his trips, and the other one would stay back to help me. If Leo stayed behind, he would run the clinic. If Leo went with the doctor, I would run it, and Makamur would take

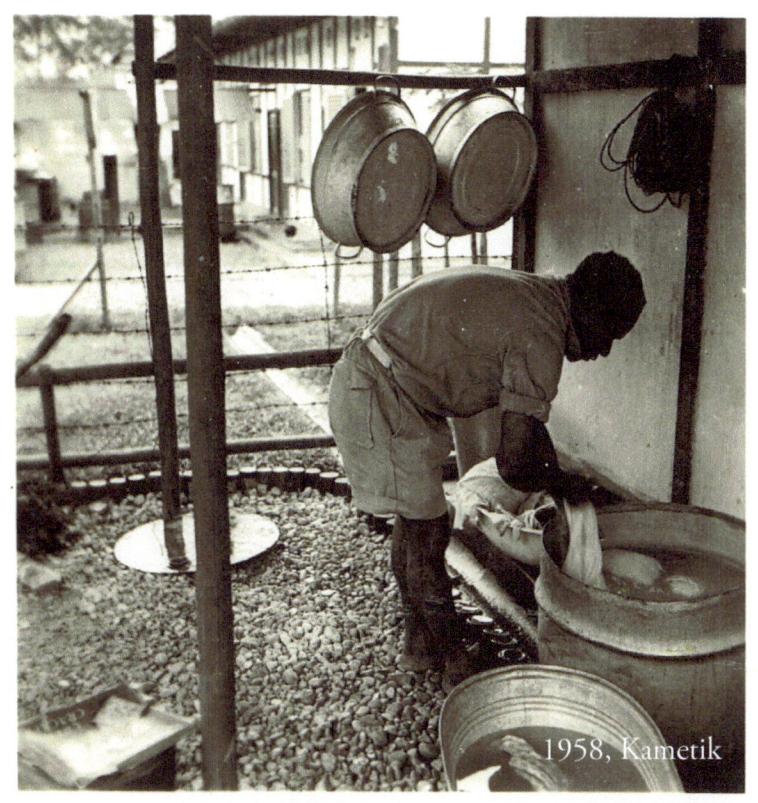

1958, Kametik

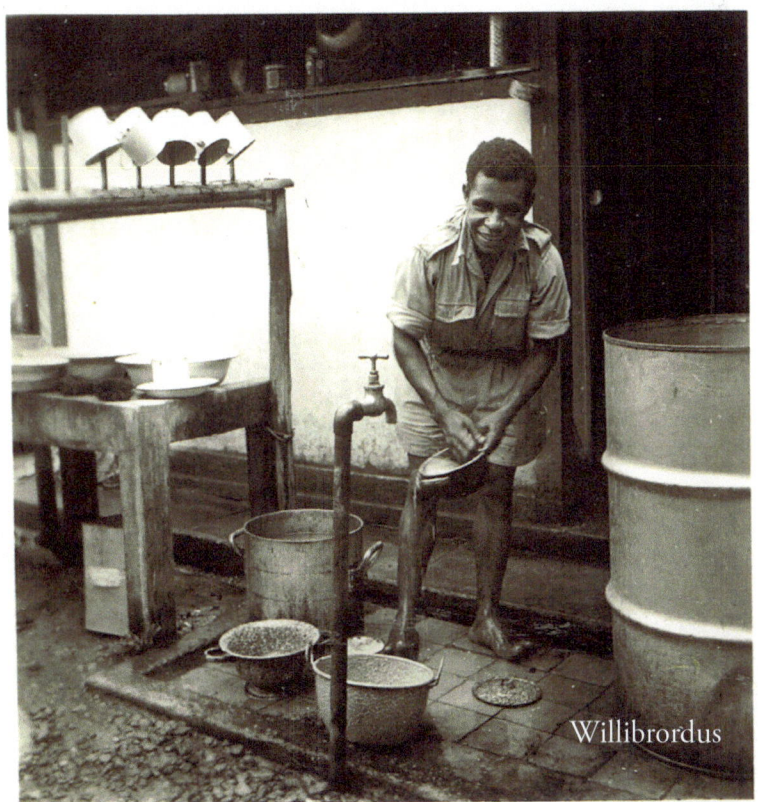

Willibrordus

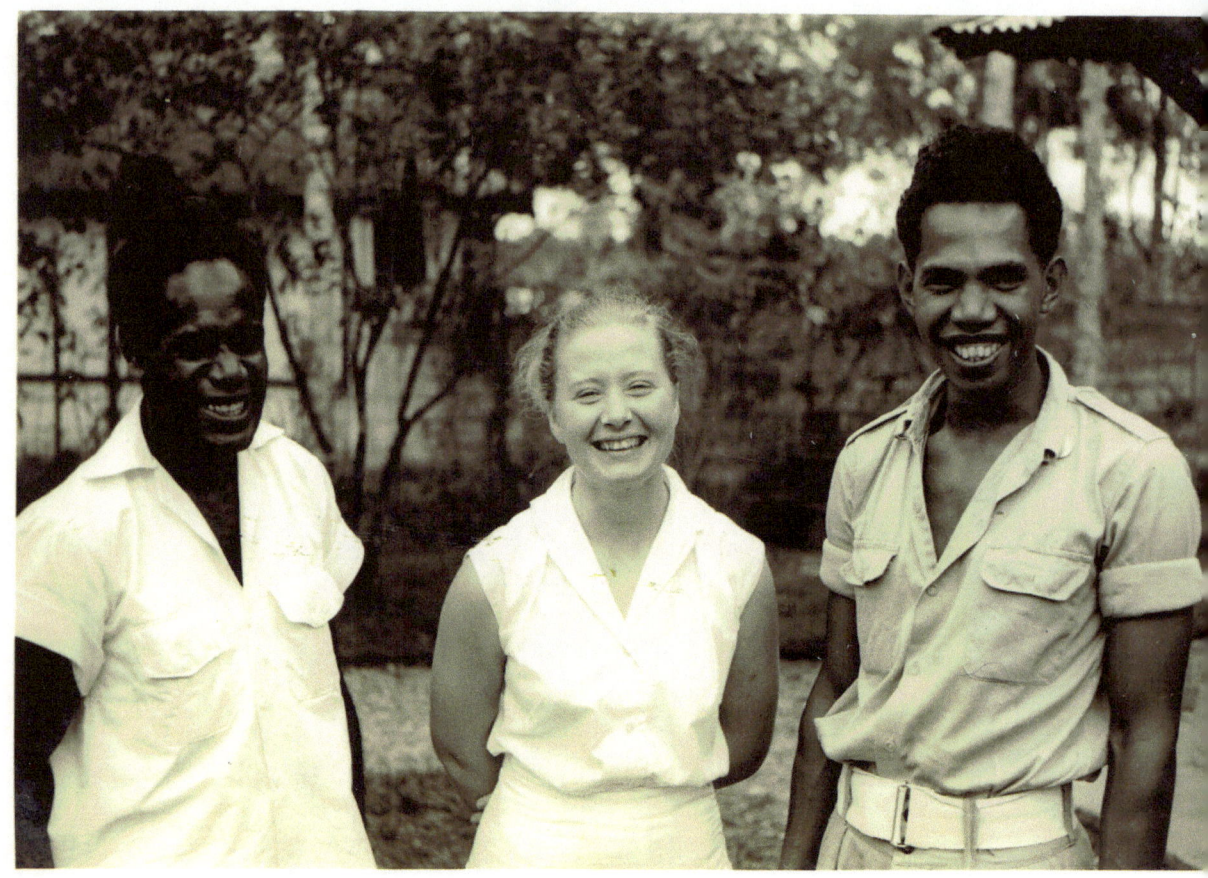

1958, Makamur, me, and Leo

care of the hospital patients.

The doctor's surveys would concentrate on the most prominent tropical diseases of the local area. We still had not much of an idea of the state of health of the people living in the jungle. Malaria was the most prevalent disease, but there was also a lot of tuberculosis and elephantiasis and kwashiorkor and framboesia.

There were also prison officers and police living in the village, and there was a small shop, run by a Chinese family. They would mainly sell rice and tinned food. We hardly saw any fresh food other than the small amount we grew.

As we were so very isolated, every department had a designated time they could have radio contact with their corresponding department in Hollandia (now Yayapura) which is the capital city of NG If we needed advice about a patient, we could talk to a doctor in Hollandia between 9 and 10 am only. Any problem at any other time? Deal with it the best you can! No flying doctor service here!

Once a week an aeroplane would come in to deliver and pick up post and sometimes bring or fetch a passenger. It would only stay for an hour.

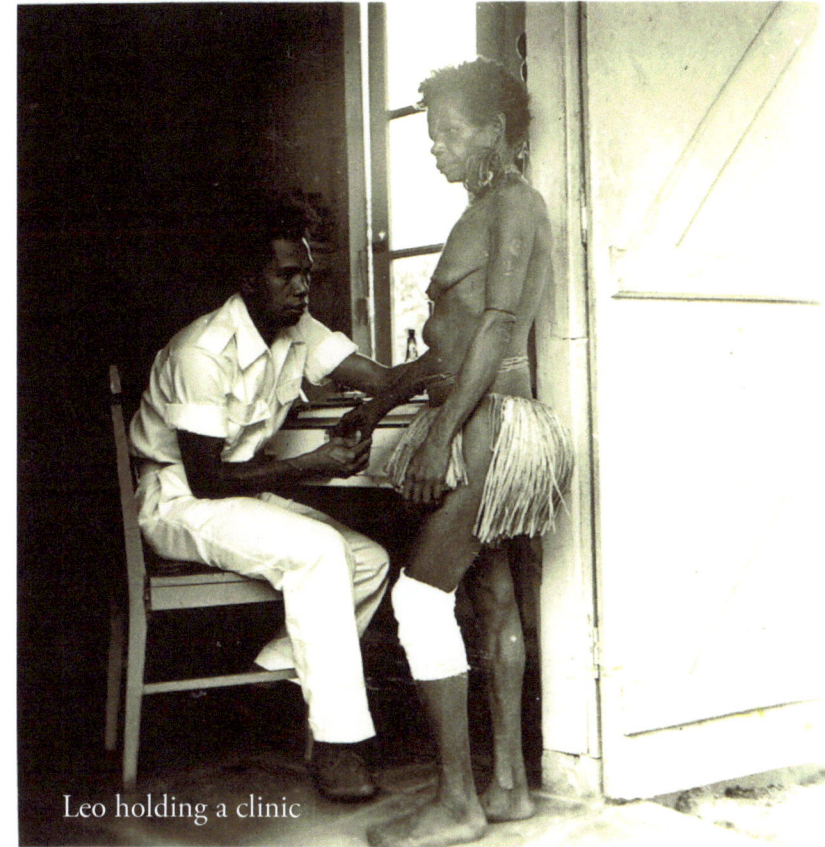
Leo holding a clinic

The nurse I replaced flew out a week after my arrival. So, we had only one week to hand over, in which time I had to get as much information as possible. It had been arranged that her furniture will get picked up when mine arrived as each nurse has their own furniture. Nurse Volkers had been here for two years and was glad to be leaving.

Some very important people I must mention here are the missionaries. There are two Dutch priests and a lovely young nun called Sister Caroline. There are also a few Papuan novices.

Sister Caroline is not only working at the school as a teacher but also looks after the meals of the priests and has offered to cook my meals as well at a very reasonable price. I accept gratefully as I have no kitchen, so I would have to cook on a primus stove or over an open fire, which is where Willibrordus cooks the food for the patients. This way at least, I get a cooked meal every day and can concentrate on my job.

Fortunately, I am not a fussy eater, so the lack of fresh food never bothered me. As far as fruits go, there were always bananas, sometimes green which were cooked as vegetables. We had a very large Jackfruit tree in front of the hospital. The fruits are so large that one fruit would feed all patients and staff and visitors. I used to love it! Then there was one other fruit called suursack. I don't know it by its English name and it is hard to describe. When ripe it is very soft, and the flesh is sour and runny like yoghurt. High in vitamin C, and very nice!

Our dinner usually existed of tinned meat or fish, rice and a vegetable called kangun. It grows wild in areas where there is enough water, so, along a stream or river. We sometimes got sweet potatoes or batates, a kind of local potato. I did miss a proper potato after a while. The shop sold tinned potatoes, but I did not like them. Rice would have to do.

Pity that pasta was not fashionable in those days because that would have made a very nice change from rice every day.

The first few days went by in a haze. I suffered from the heat and information overload.

My colleague was drinking hot black coffee all day. Remember, we only had a small fridge run on paraffin for some medications and no room for cold drinks.

Once I was on my own, I started to take stock of what we had by the way of drugs, instruments, bandages etc. I was quite surprised at the number of instruments. Syringes of all sizes, but no autoclave, so everything had to be boiled in a pot on a primus stove.

I noticed we had very little linen. A few sheets and no more than six towels. When I queried that, I was told that the natives did not use sheets and if we had a European patient they would bring their own, so what we had was adequate.

I tried to learn as much Indonesian as I could in my spare time as well as on the job as that was the only way to communicate with the patients. Dr Henk had to go away on a survey after a month. By now I knew the name of the different body parts in Indonesian. I used my Dutch-Indonesian dictionary a lot. That became my treasured Bible.

When Henk left, I was quietly confident that I could cope. The people were all so friendly, and I loved the life in a small place in the middle of nowhere.

Strangely enough, I was never homesick! I would write home every week, and although the post took a while, we all looked forward to the plane on a Wednesday and our post. There was always a letter from home and often one from one of my friends, especially from Els, who had moved to France and was working for Abbe Pierre, a priest, caring for the poor. She was a volunteer, and it was there she met her husband, who worked with her for a while. They married and settled in Paris after some time.

Henk's wife Loes often came over to have coffee with me when her husband was away, and she encouraged me to come and play volleyball in town every day at 5 pm. I did whenever I could. If there was an emergency at the hospital someone would call me, as it was very close.

I also enjoyed my visits with sister Caroline. I used to bring my rantang back to the mission. A rantang is a holder with three or four containers in which my dinner was delivered to the hospital by one of the novices. They would come and collect it, but I enjoyed taking it back as sister Caroline became such a good friend and we used to have a glass of lemon drink together.

Was I ever scared? No, not really. But, there was one time we had a very severe thunderstorm at night. It was so close, that I was sure someone's house would have been hit. I was really scared then! When I ventured outside the next morning, several big trees close to the hospital had been uprooted, but no houses had been hit. The heavy rain had prevented any fires. Thank God, everyone was alright.

Once, while the doctor was away, one young government employee came to see me with a terrible toothache. He begged me to take the tooth out. Henk was not due back for another two weeks. I knew we had a full set of dental pliers, and we had the anaesthetic, so I injected him and found the right pliers and took the tooth out. He was ever so grateful! And I was so glad we had had a lecture on extractions by a dentist in our six week course. I gave him some Panadol, and he was fine. As there was only one aeroplane coming on a Wednesday, we had to deal with any emergency the best we could.

Loes and Henk had a housemaid called Suzanna, who was pregnant. When she went into labour, she came to the hospital for the delivery. However, the labour did not progress. The baby went into distress, and Henk decided that she needed a caesarean section. Wow! This was huge! Henk was a GP, with an interest in Chirurgy, but had never done a caesarean. We were not equipped for major surgery.

He told me that I would have to give the anaesthetic. I had seen while working in the theatre during my training, how ether anaesthetic was given; but I was only observing, and that was a few years ago. Anyway, we had no choice. I went looking for a Schimmelbush mask and ether and chloroform. Yes, that was all there. Now the instruments! Did we have all that was needed? Yes, we did! But no autoclave! So, I had to boil the instruments in a big pot on the primus stove.

One needs drapes, and big swabs and all we had sterile was a small tin of 4x4s (small gauzes).

We decided that we could iron the six towels we had and iron some sheets with an iron on the outside fire. At last, everything was ready to go. Suzanna was excellent and trusted us implicitly, so no panic there. Henk had read up on how to do a caesarean. Leo was to assist Henk and Makamur would stand by in case we needed anything.

I had given Suzanna a pre-med. And she was getting sleepy. I started by putting chloroform on the mask slowly. After a short while, the patient went into the exaltation stadium, which means, she began to go into spasms. Henk panicked. What is happening? What are you doing? I told him, "don't worry! This is normal. You just have to wait. It's only the exaltation stadium." How I remembered that I don't know, but I continued with dripping ether now, and when the patient was relaxed, I told Henk that he could begin.

The baby was born within a few minutes and fortunately started to cry almost immediately. It was a girl! After the placenta was born, the patient was stitched up and moved to a bed. We all heaved a big sigh of relief! It seemed the operation had been a success!

Henk went back to his book to check if he had done everything right and suddenly called out, "oh my God!",

"What is it, Henk?" I asked.

"I think I have stitched the bladder to the uterus! Did you see it?" He asked, bewildered.

I replied, "no I am sorry, I did not watch you, I was watching Suzanna and the baby".

Henk was very worried. Should we open her up again? I suggested not to do anything and wait if Suzanna was passing urine first. He implored me to call him immediately day or night when Suzanna urinated. I slept that first night next to Suzanna, and at 2 am she wanted to wee. I got her onto a bedpan and surprise, surprise, she passed a beautiful yellow wee, without a trace of blood. What a relief! As promised I ran to Henk's house with the bedpan and knocked on his bedroom window. Henk come and look! And we both danced around with the bedpan laughing with glee.

All was well, and mother and baby did well.

One day a couple brought a very sick looking baby to the clinic. The child was very undernourished, and the parents were incredibly anxious. They had walked for three days and were not from this area. They did not speak the local language, and none of the staff could communicate with them. At first, we could not diagnose what was wrong with the baby but treated her for dehydration as she was vomiting and had diarrhoea. She did not respond. She would have been about nine months old but only weighed 3,050 grams.

After a few days, the parents wanted to go home as they had other children at home.

They indicated that they wanted to leave the baby with us. So, I now was a foster parent!!

As I could not pronounce the little girl's name, I renamed her Elsje, after my best friend Els in France.

Elsje was a lovely little girl. I grew very fond of her. She was eventually diagnosed with coeliac disease, not a very well-known condition in the 50s.

The staple food of the local people was sago and batates, and it was hard for us to find any food that Elsje would be able to tolerate when back with her

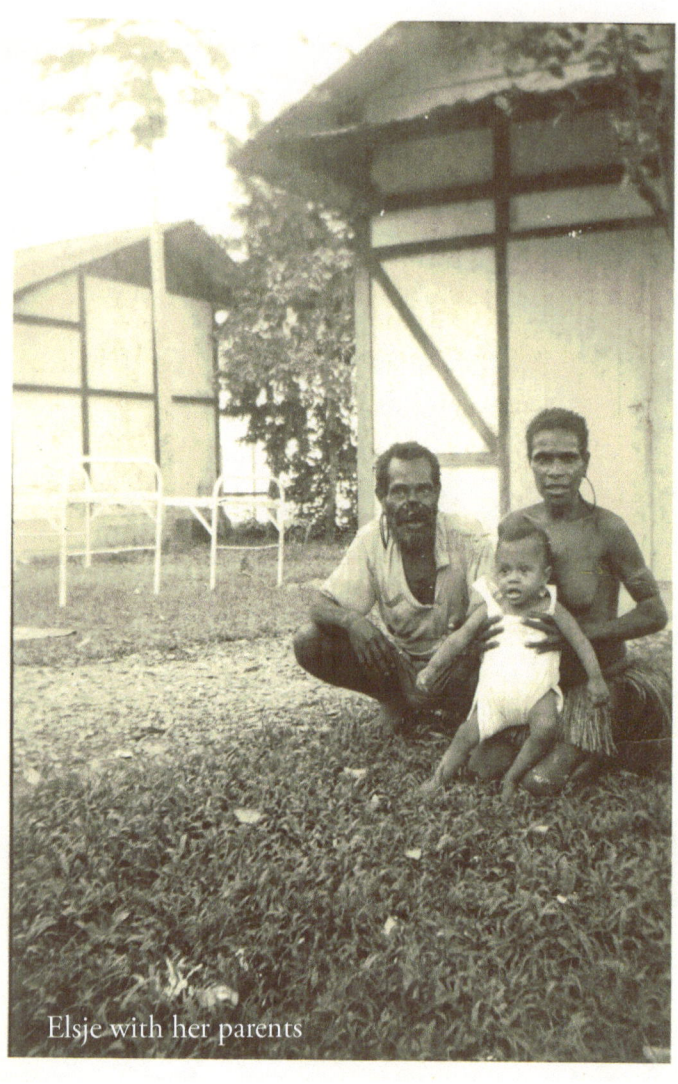
Elsje with her parents

parents. She responded well to rice and mung beans which are high in protein.

After three months her parents came back to fetch her. They were so pleased to see how well she looked. They wanted to take her home of course. We tried to tell them that she could not eat the sago or batates anymore. We showed them how to cook rice and mung beans and gave them a large bag of each to take home. We told them to come back for more when the food was finished. How much they understood I do not know. Language can be such a barrier. They left, and we never saw them again. It broke my heart to see them go.

Another case I found very hard to deal with, was a woman with advanced tuberculosis. I had started to treat her while Dr Henk was away.

When he came home and saw her in the ward, he told me I should not have admitted her. She was too far gone and could not be treated successfully, as that would take years and he knew she would not come back for medication once she felt a bit better. In the meantime, she would infect dozens of people, so the sooner she died, the better for all. I found that so hard, but had to admit that it made sense. So very reluctantly I had to tell her she could go home (to die really). Sometimes one has to be cruel to be kind.

That was a hard lesson to learn.

After having been in Tanah Merah for quite a few months, I asked Henk if maybe I could go on a survey instead of him. He gave it some thought and came back to me saying, "O.K. You can go on a week's survey of some villages along the river Digul. You can take Makamur with you, who is from this area and some porters, as you will have to walk from the river to the villages that are three to four hours walk from the riverfront." By now I knew enough Indonesian to hold a clinic in each village.

Every village has a passangrahan (a guesthouse) to be used by any passing patrol, be it a doctor, police officer, or government official. It's an empty house. You bring your bedding; which used to be a mosquito net, blanket and sleeping mat. Also, food and tea or coffee, along with anything else you might like. It made a welcome change for me from life in Tanah Merah, and I found it very interesting to see how the people in the jungle lived.

I thoroughly enjoyed the trip, and the birdlife was fantastic! We saw many birds of paradise and toucans. The walking was not easy, especially as you always had leeches getting into your jungle boots. One could get them off with a burning cigarette. (I did smoke then).

I was very grateful for the porters as I did not have to carry anything. Crossing the occasional river was tricky as there would be a slippery tree trunk laid across. I would walk between two porters who would each hold my hand, so I would not slip and fall in.

I enjoyed the trip, and the people were always very friendly and respectful. Although very primitive in many ways, they had inherent decency. For instance, if I needed to wee while we were peddling on the river I only had to look at the shore and they would ask, "do you want to stop sister?" They would drop me at a convenient spot, peddle on a few hundred yards and then come back for me. As the guesthouse never had any doors and I had to wash, one person would post himself in front of the door facing outwards, and I could strip and wash and they would never look back. Some villages had a river right through the village, and then you would have a bathroom. They would stick a large bamboo stick into the river and build a small shed around the other end, and you had a lovely shower with running water.

It was at this time that the oil companies started to explore New Guinea for oil. A Dutch company had based itself on a houseboat on the river Digul close to Tanah Merah. They had their headquarters in Sorong and maintained contact with Sorong by Catalina plane. Much like fly in fly out, here in Western Australia these days. Some of the young men would come to the clinic with minor ailments, and one of them became quite a regular visitor. He invited me to go to lunch on the houseboat one Sunday and was to pick me up at midday. He came by motorboat and after a lovely meal of fresh meat and all things not available in the local Chinese shop. We ate beautiful potatoes that I had missed a lot. Then, he took me back and asked if he could see me again. He was due for a break in Sorong for ten days and asked if he could get me anything. I declined, but when he came back, he brought me a record player with some lovely records and invited me again to lunch the next Sunday on the houseboat.

This time a helicopter landed in front of the hospital at midday to pick me up. Wow! Of course, I was excited, and it was then that I realised he was trying to impress me!

Will was ten years older than me and of Dutch-Indonesian descent. I was flattered by the attention and did like him a lot. Over the next few months, he showered me with presents: Chanel number 5 and a watch, among other things. He would always come back from Sorong with a surprise.

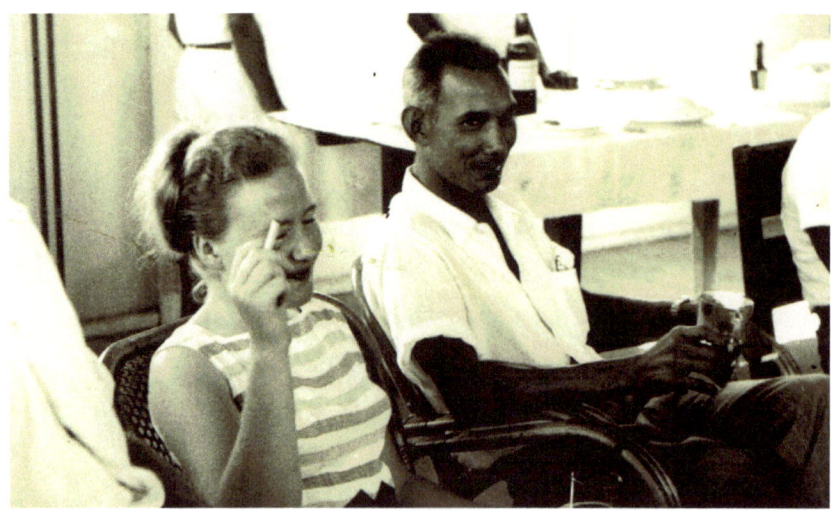

Lunch on the houseboat, me and Will

But, there was one thing about him that worried me. He was very possessive and jealous. He did not like me to talk to anyone and would get angry if I was a few minutes later back from volleyball or the shop than expected. Otherwise, he treated me like a queen, so when after about four months of seeing him, he asked me to marry him, I said yes.

I asked my sister Riet to send me a wedding dress and started preparations for a small wedding. The priest had met Will and was pleased that I was marrying a Catholic in his church.

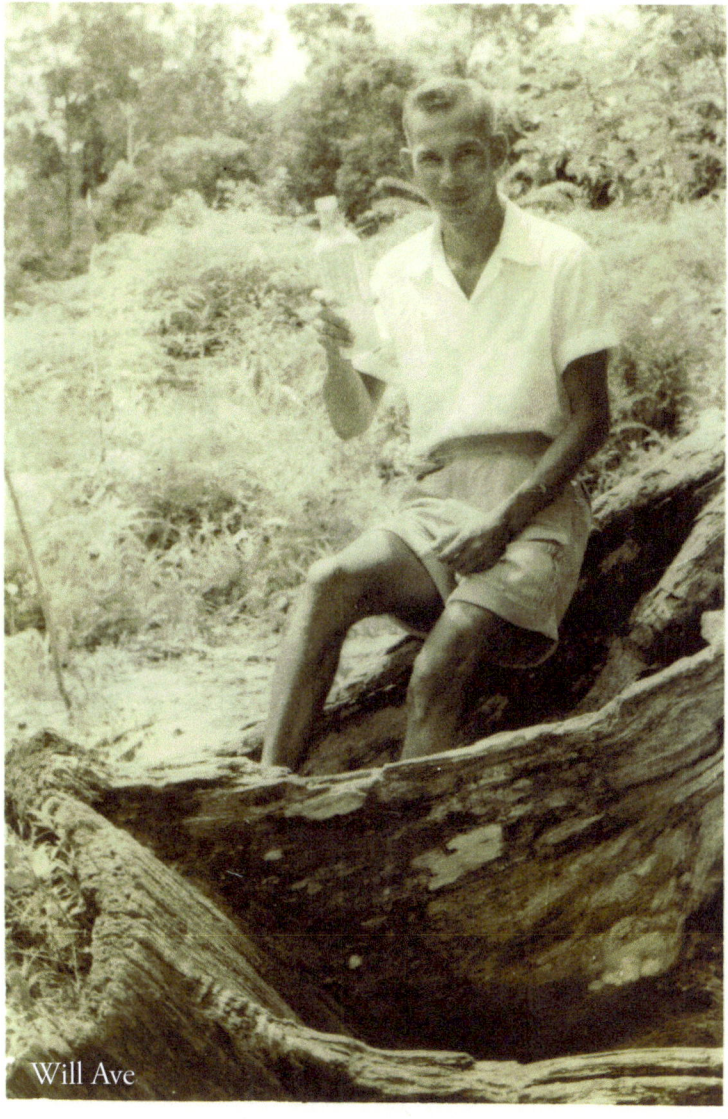
Will Ave

I put some notices around the village on trees inviting people to attend the service and reception.

Will was on leave in Sorong, when ten days before the wedding I woke up in the middle of the night and thought, 'Oh my God! What am I going to do? This is a big mistake!' It was suddenly obvious to me that I was infatuated, but not really in love with Will. I got up and tore all the notices off the trees. I felt awful for Will but knew I could not go through with it. Unfortunately, I could not ring him, so the next morning I sent a telegram telling him not to come and wait for my letter.

Frans and Henk came to see me in the morning having seen the notices taken down. When I told them of my decision, they said, "thank God! We did not think you should marry him. So we are glad that it is not too late."

I was quite indignant. If they all thought that, then why did none of them talk to me about it? "You all know I am here all alone without any family and you thought I was making a mistake and did not say anything! Thanks very much!" "O.K. We probably should have talked to you, and we are sorry. Is there anything we can do now?" They replied.

I said, "yes there is. I have given notice, and I would like to keep working. There has already a replacement for me been appointed, but, maybe you could sort this out for me?" They said, "leave it with us".

Of course, Will did come, and I had a few challenging days with him. He was devastated, and I felt so guilty, but I knew that it was the right thing to do.

The new nurse arrived, and I got a transfer to Hollandia.

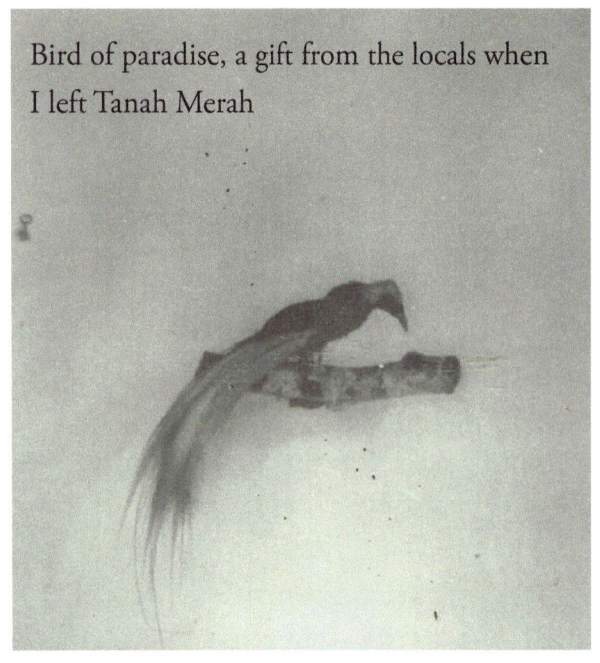

Bird of paradise, a gift from the locals when I left Tanah Merah

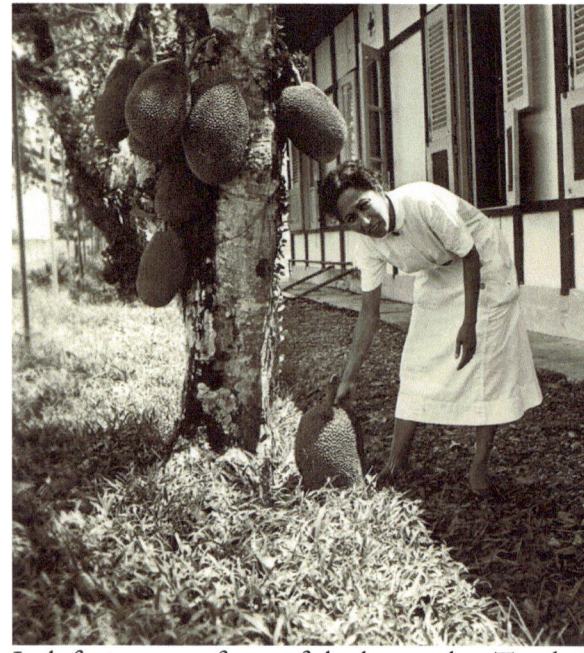

Jack fruit tree in front of the hospital in Tanah Merah with the nurse who replaced me

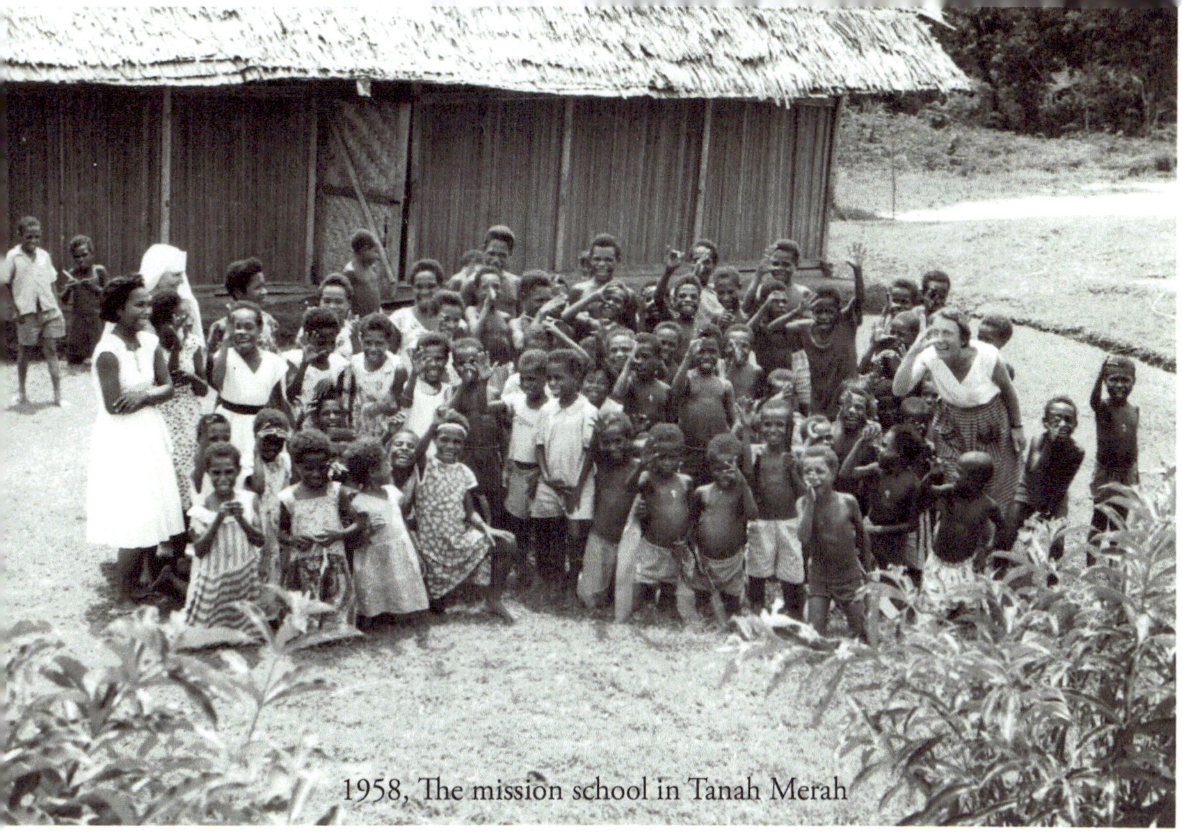

1958, The mission school in Tanah Merah

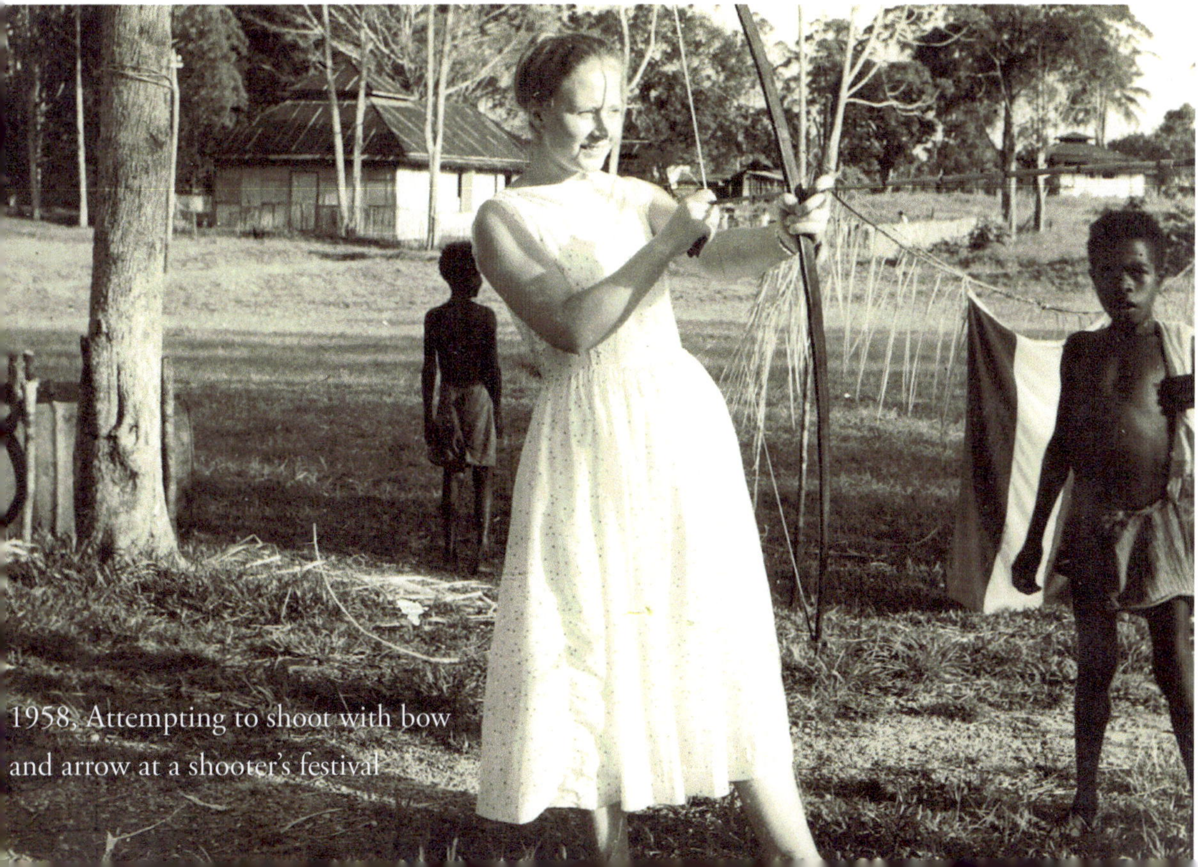

1958, Attempting to shoot with bow
and arrow at a shooter's festival

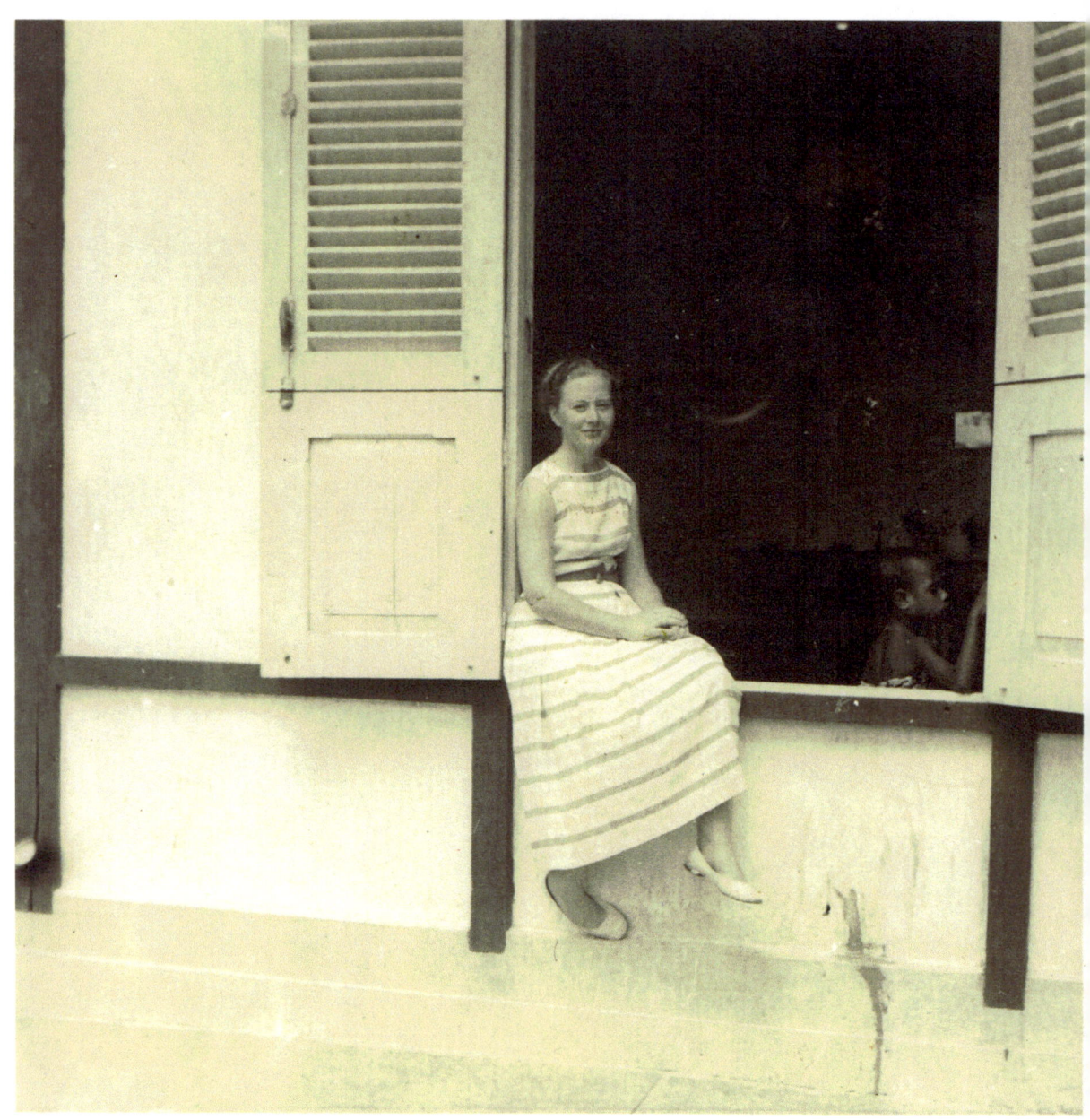

At home in front of the window

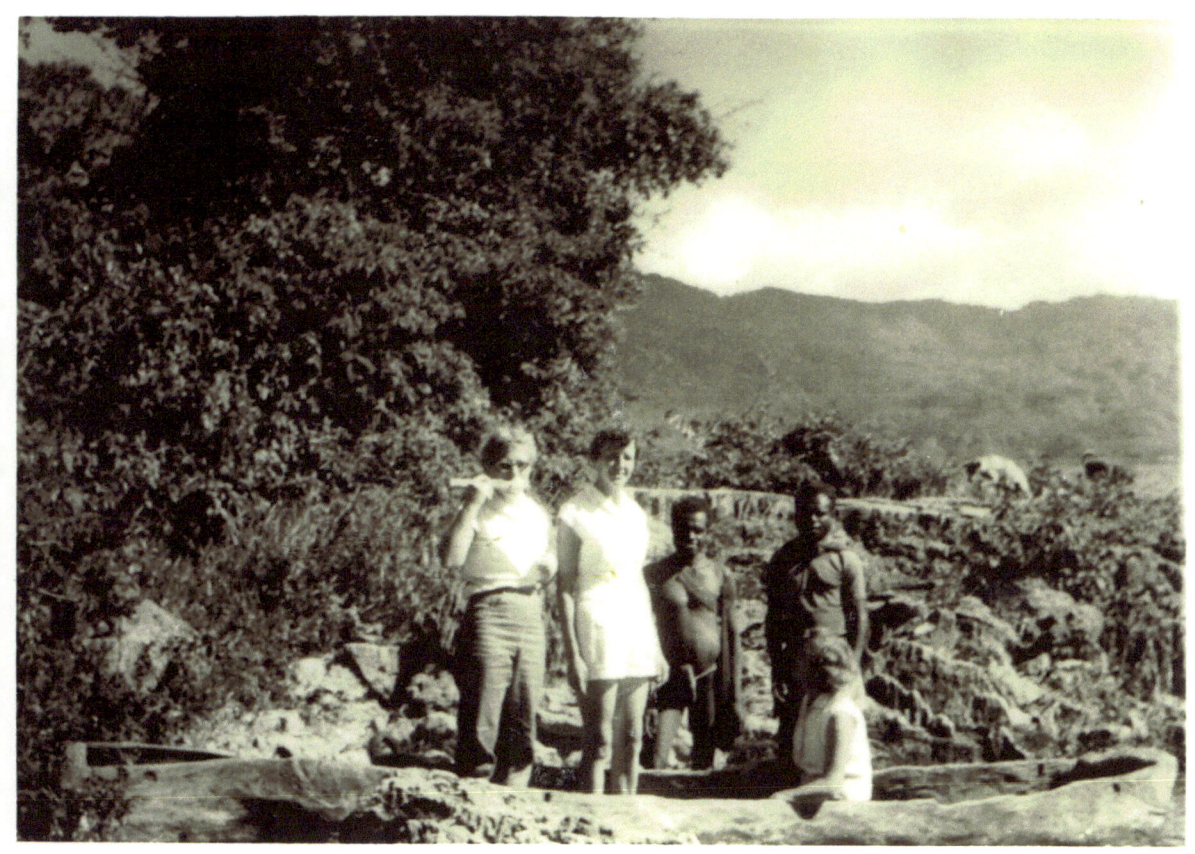
Sucking on a piece of sugar beet

HOLLANDIA

It was quite a change to be working in a relatively new and well-equipped hospital again. I enjoyed having colleagues again. Everyone seemed to be riding scooters although there were only fifty kilometres of sealed roads. I very soon bought myself a 125 cc Vespa scooter and enjoyed a bit of social life.

Lake Sentani was thirty kilometres away and used for swimming and water-skiing, so I learned to ski.

Being close to the ocean it was not as hot here as in Tanah Merah. The hospital was not air conditioned, but when you were on night duty, you got an air conditioned room to sleep in, which was nice. I did enjoy night duty here. After working at the hospital for about eight months, I was asked if I was interested in coming and working for the KSB, which was the mother and child service. This was run in conjunction with the mission, so was church-based and government supported. They were in need of a nurse that could speak Indonesian, and my name had come up.

I was delighted as this was a much wanted job, and I would have to move to Hollandia Binnen.

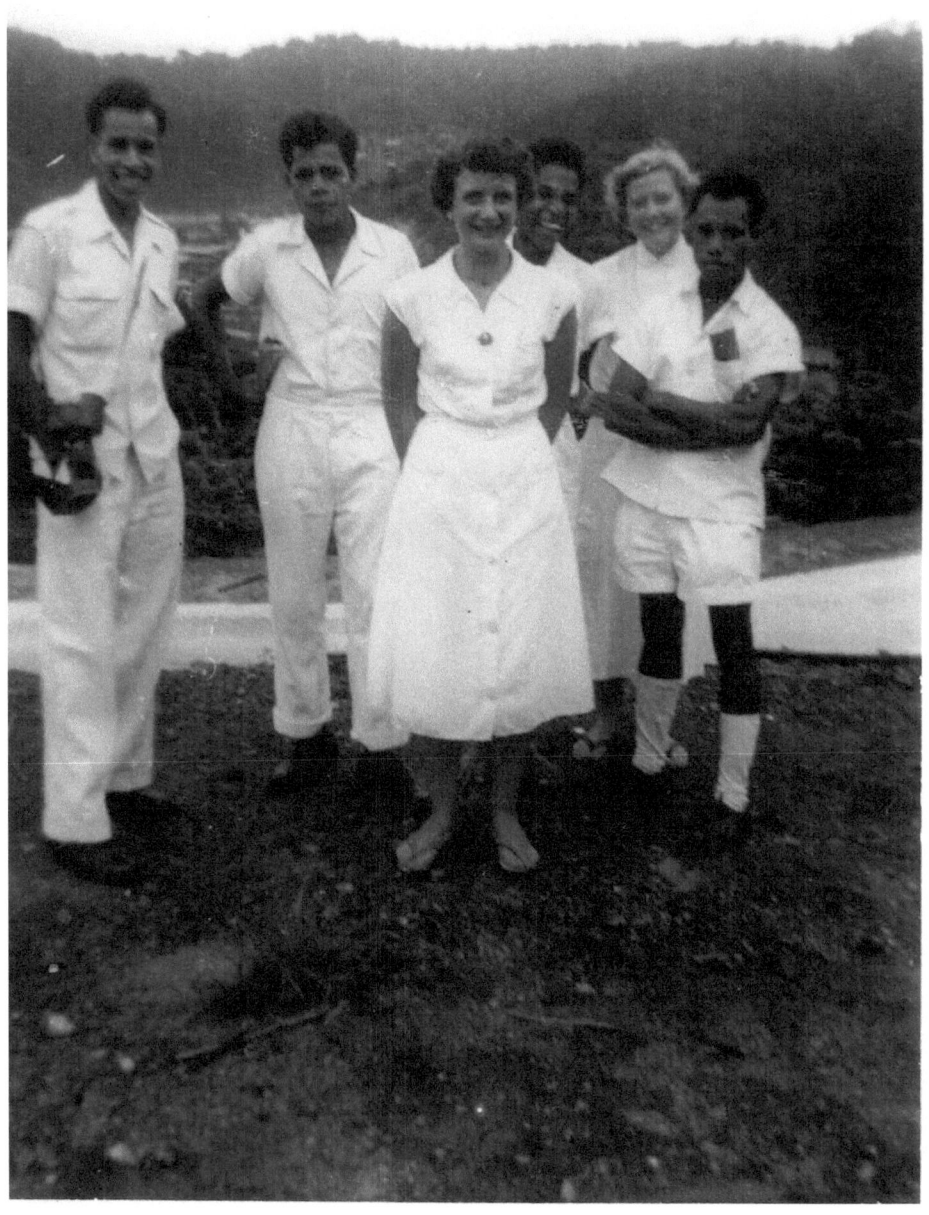
Jopie Engbrecht and me with some of the staff from Hollandia hospital

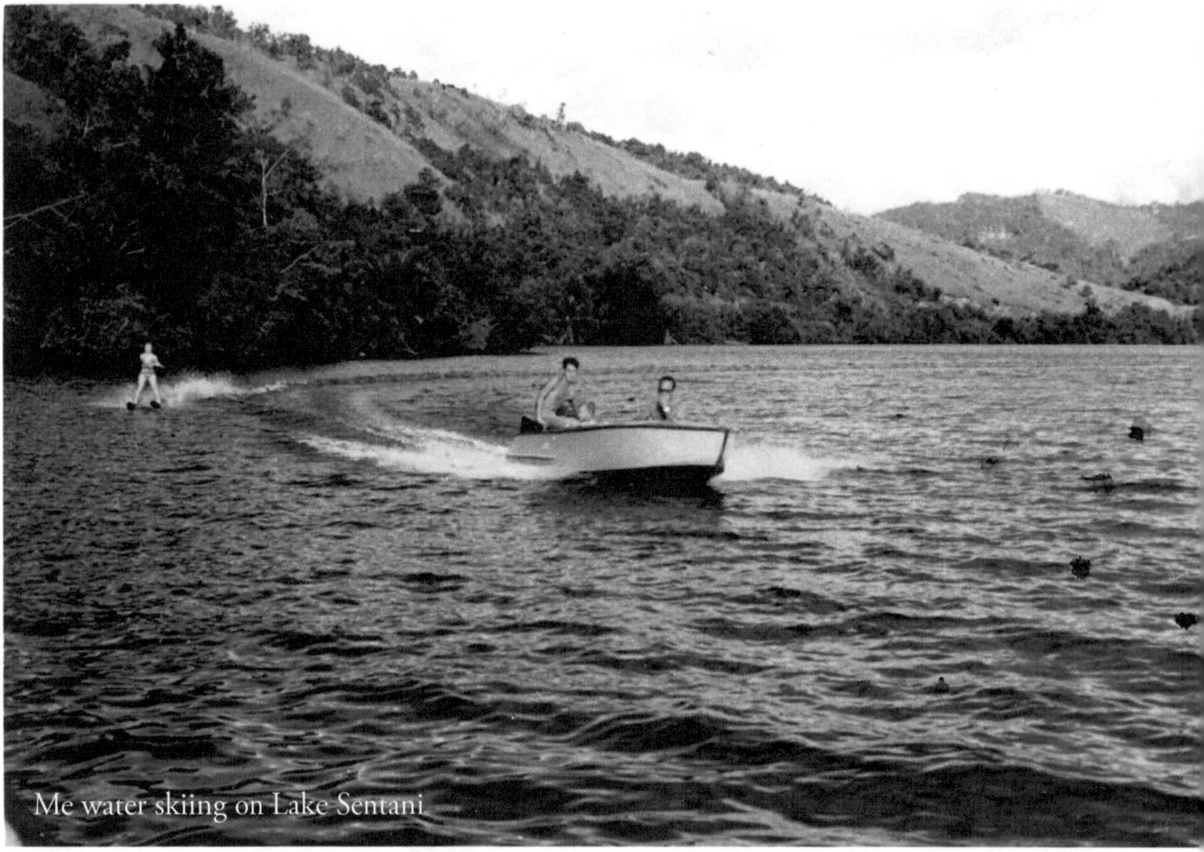

Me water skiing on Lake Sentani

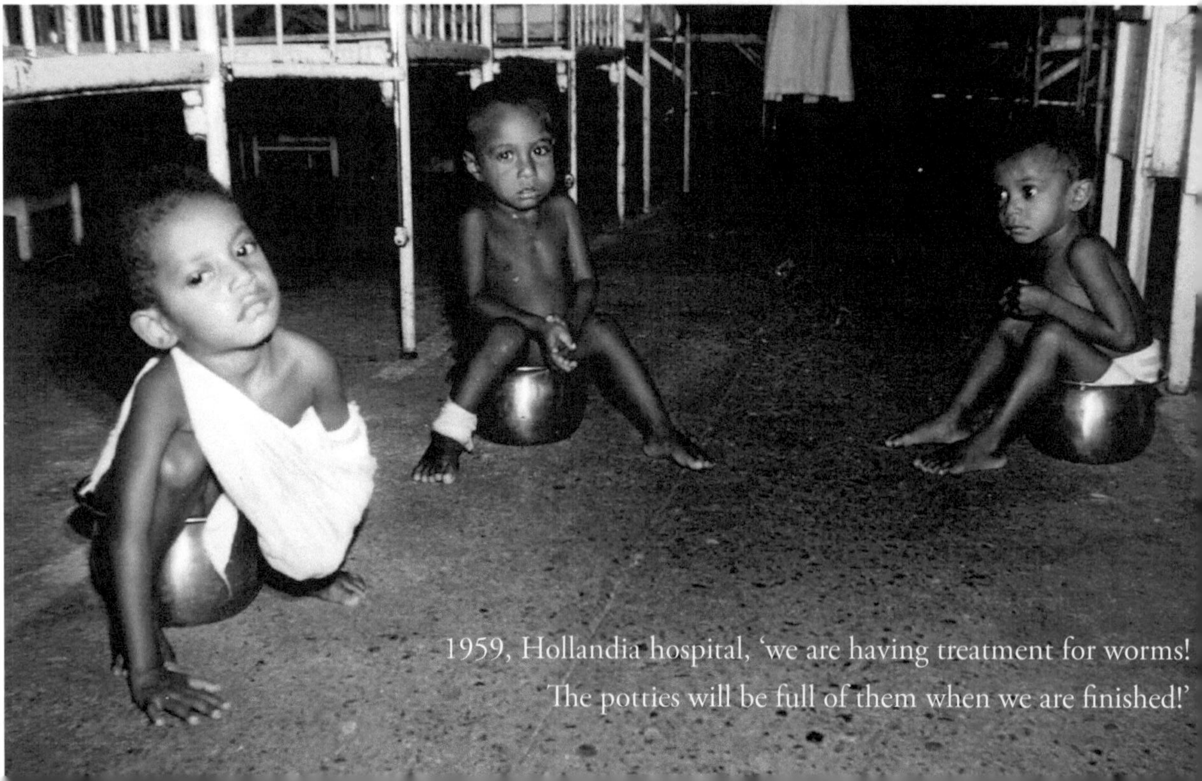

1959, Hollandia hospital, 'we are having treatment for worms! The potties will be full of them when we are finished!'

This service trained local girls to be health workers. The course took two years, and in that time, they would learn how to run a clinic for babies and toddlers. Also, to do a routine delivery and refer any cases of concern to hospital. After the successful training, the health worker would be placed in the centre village of her district and travel to each village to hold clinics for pregnant women as well as children, weighing them and giving advice on nutrition etc.

I first had to learn to drive a V.W. Kombi as we took the trainees to various points in Sentani and Hollandia to hold clinics and do some home deliveries or if needed take the patient to the hospital. We would give nutritional advice and always carried milk powder which we gave out as there was a significant protein deficiency in the diet of the locals.

After a few months of training the girls, I was asked to be a supervisor of the girls, working in the district. I would be away three weeks at the time. My area would be along the coast between Hollandia and Sarmi. Four girls were

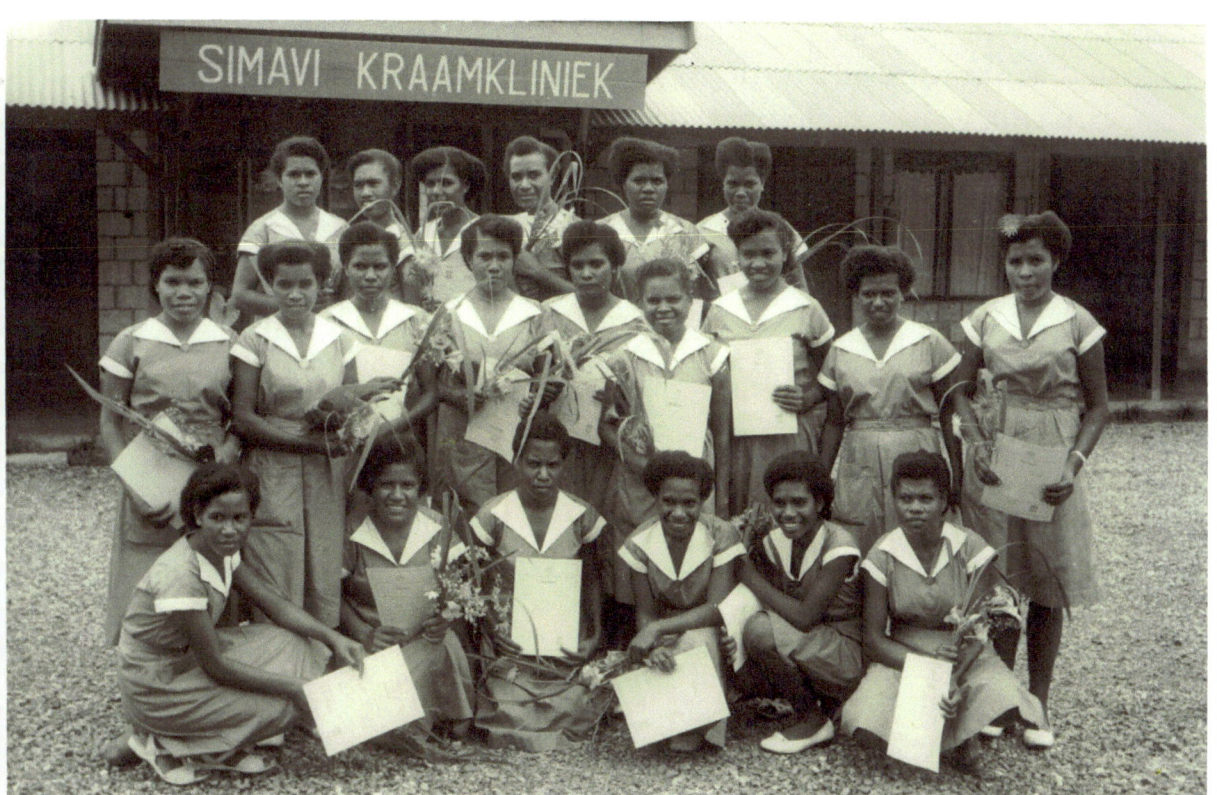

1960, Graduation of a class of health workers in Hollandia

working along this strip. Each would have the care of three or four villages.

For a village to qualify for a health worker, the village would have to provide housing and transport for the health worker. Here transportation was a prauw with a crew. The Kapala Kampong (head of the village) would appoint the men each time, so they all took turns. The prauws had outriggers as the ocean could be a bit rough sometimes. They are very steady, and the men are all excellent seamen and good fishermen too!

The first health worker would meet me in her first village, and after working there, we would move on to the next village. I was there to support the health worker, answer any questions and teach wherever needed. The people were always pleased to see us and keen to learn. I used to carry a projector (run on paraffin) and screen and show slides of whatever was appropriate at the time. Educational always, but the whole village used to come out to watch and listen and ask questions, and I discovered that I enjoyed teaching. "Sister, are you going to show a film tonight?" was music to my ears.

I also learned a lot from them as they had their own way of treating different ailments and had done so for thousands of years some with good results. For instance, they used the young leaves of a pawpaw tree to treat malaria with a good result; it was drunk as a tea.

Many of the villages had an Indonesian teacher, and often I was invited to spend the night in their home. They were always so hospitable. I would leave them some of my provisions as a thank you. Coffee was always very well received, and so was corned beef. The next morning we would move on to the next village. The sea could be a bit rough, and I usually enjoyed the ride, but once I remember getting seasick. I felt awful! It was then that I noticed we were suddenly going much faster and when I asked why, I was told, "there is a turtle we want to catch!" They caught it, tied it to the boat and again started to row very fast. Another turtle was captured and when we arrived at the village, I realised I was not seasick anymore. Mind over matter! The chase had taken over, and I had not been feeling sick anymore.

That night I had my first taste of turtle meat and eggs as one of the turtles was a female with about thirty eggs inside. This was such a treat for the whole village, who typically live on fish and very occasionally some pork. I found the meat very tasty, a bit between chicken and goat meat.

Pigs are very important in the culture of the Papua. They would roam freely in the village and eat whatever they could find. If they saw you going to the toilet they would follow you in the hope you would do 'number two' and eat that too. Women would sometimes breastfeed a little piglet as well as her baby if the piglet was a runt and did not feed well at the sow.

The health workers did an outstanding job and were respected in their villages as the people started to see an improvement in the health of the children if and when they followed her advice regarding hygiene and nutrition. I would continue to carry lots of milk powder, and all the schoolchildren would get a drink of milk every day, which may not seem much, but at least they would get some protein and calcium.

The young mothers were taught to start supplementing their babies at four months old with a bit of kangun (wild spinach), and sago as the mother's diet was usually poor and the breastmilk, therefore, lacked nutrition. They learned how vital the colostrum is and they were taught that the old belief of colostrum being poisonous to the baby actually robbed the baby of the first most important feeds. (This belief was in some areas, not general). This was a delightful time for me in my nursing career as I felt I was making a difference. The people were eager to learn, which gave me great job satisfaction.

The WHO (World Health Organisation) did send a doctor out to New Guinea specifically to have a look of what was being done by the KSB. (Mother and Child Care), and so Dr Poortman arrived in Hollandia.

Having lived in Indonesia for many years, Dr P. spoke fluent Indonesian, and after spending a few weeks in Hollandia, he wanted to accompany me on my next field trip. I did learn a lot from him and enjoyed his company. He was a joyous person, who could enjoy the simple things in life. He seemed to be impressed with the way I was handling the job, which was nice.

When his twelve-year-old son came out from Holland for a holiday he came again with me for a week and brought his son with him. When he left to return to Holland, he gave me a travel alarm clock with a note inside saying, 'good night, where ever you are!' I have still got it.

As I usually got some time off between trips, I managed to visit the

Baliem Valley and the Wisselmeren (Wissel Lakes). Both places are in the centre of NG and only accessible by air.

The only Europeans living amongst the Papuans in these places are the missionaries. Priests as well as some nuns. A friend and I could get a lift with

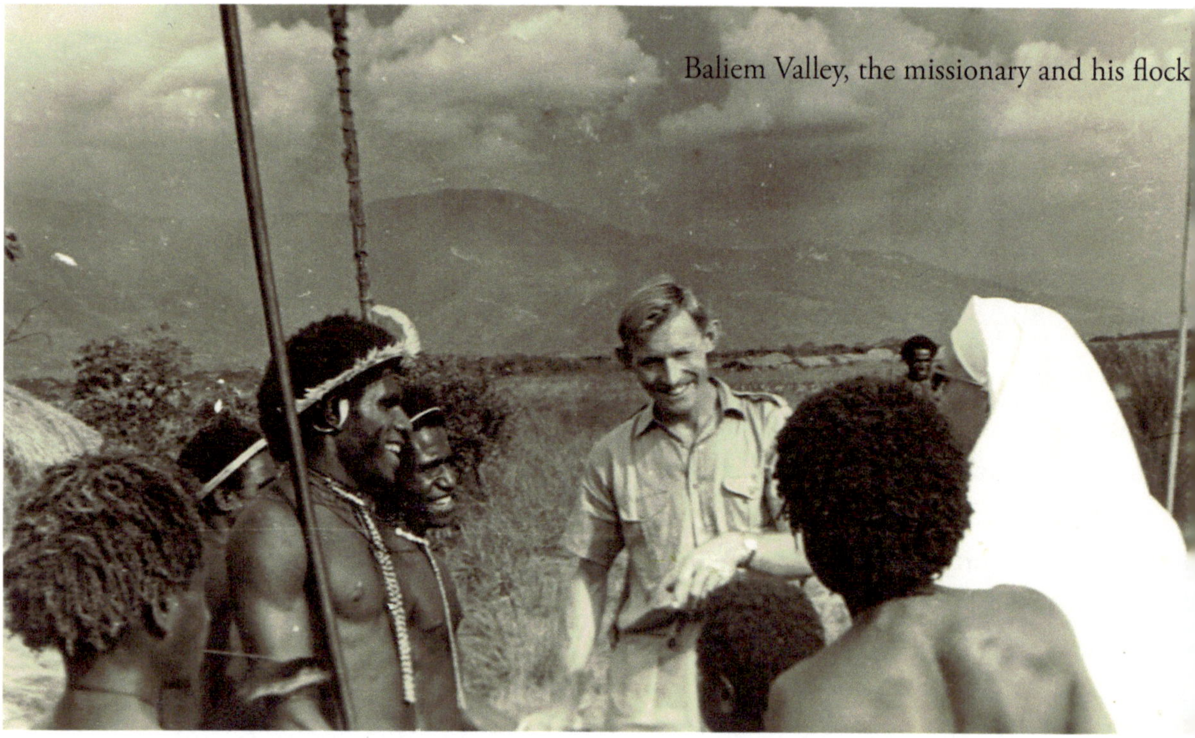

Baliem Valley, the missionary and his flock

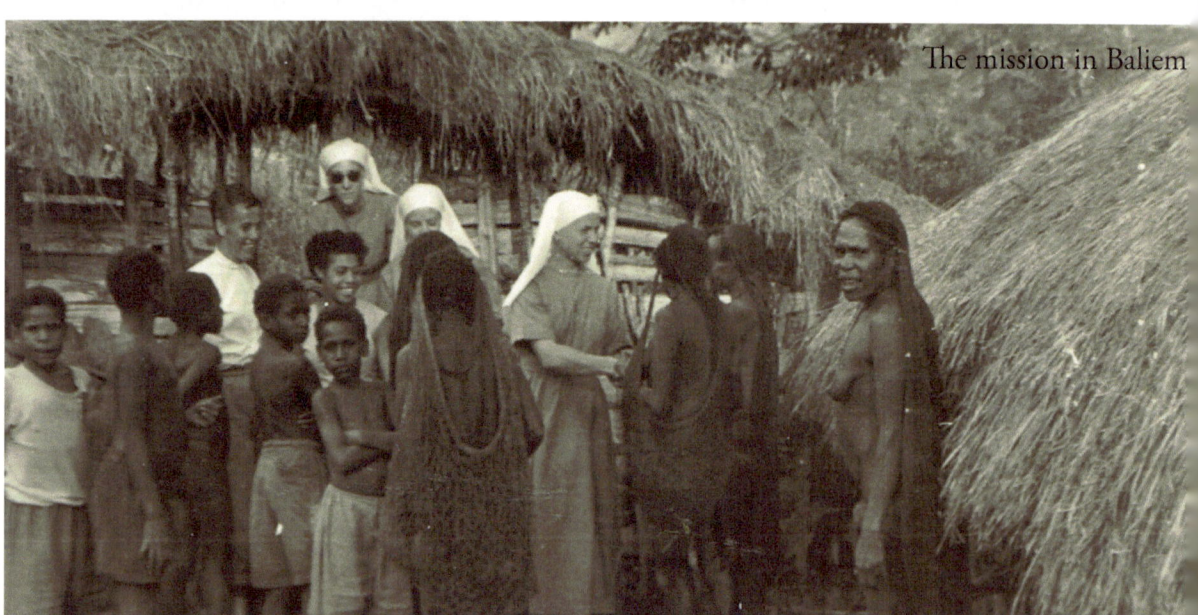

The mission in Baliem

a Cessna aeroplane that would take us to the mission, and we could stay there. The missionaries used to take us around and seemed pleased to have company. Their life was pretty lonely. The nuns were very adventurous and would do things like crossing a large river on a simple raft.

In some isolated villages we were the first white women the natives had seen, and they wanted to touch us. Our legs where of especially great interest to the women as they have mostly very skinny legs.

In the past, most Dutch personnel would get six months leave after a three-year contract and then sign on for another three years. However, when my three-year contract was coming to an end, I was told I could not renew my contract but could stay for another six months if I wished.

The Indonesian government had decided that NG was an excellent place to send some people from the very overpopulated island of Java, and maybe there were some minerals after all; as the Dutch were exploring all over the island with some success. My friend Ida Boerstra whose contract was running out at the same time as mine decided to stay, as did I. We would then travel back to Holland together instead of flying. Ida did the same work as I did, and we had become terrific friends.

So, after our last six months, we had to leave, and it was with heavy hearts that we said goodbye to all our girls and the people we had grown to love so much. I knew that I was leaving a country and its people that I would always remember with great affection.

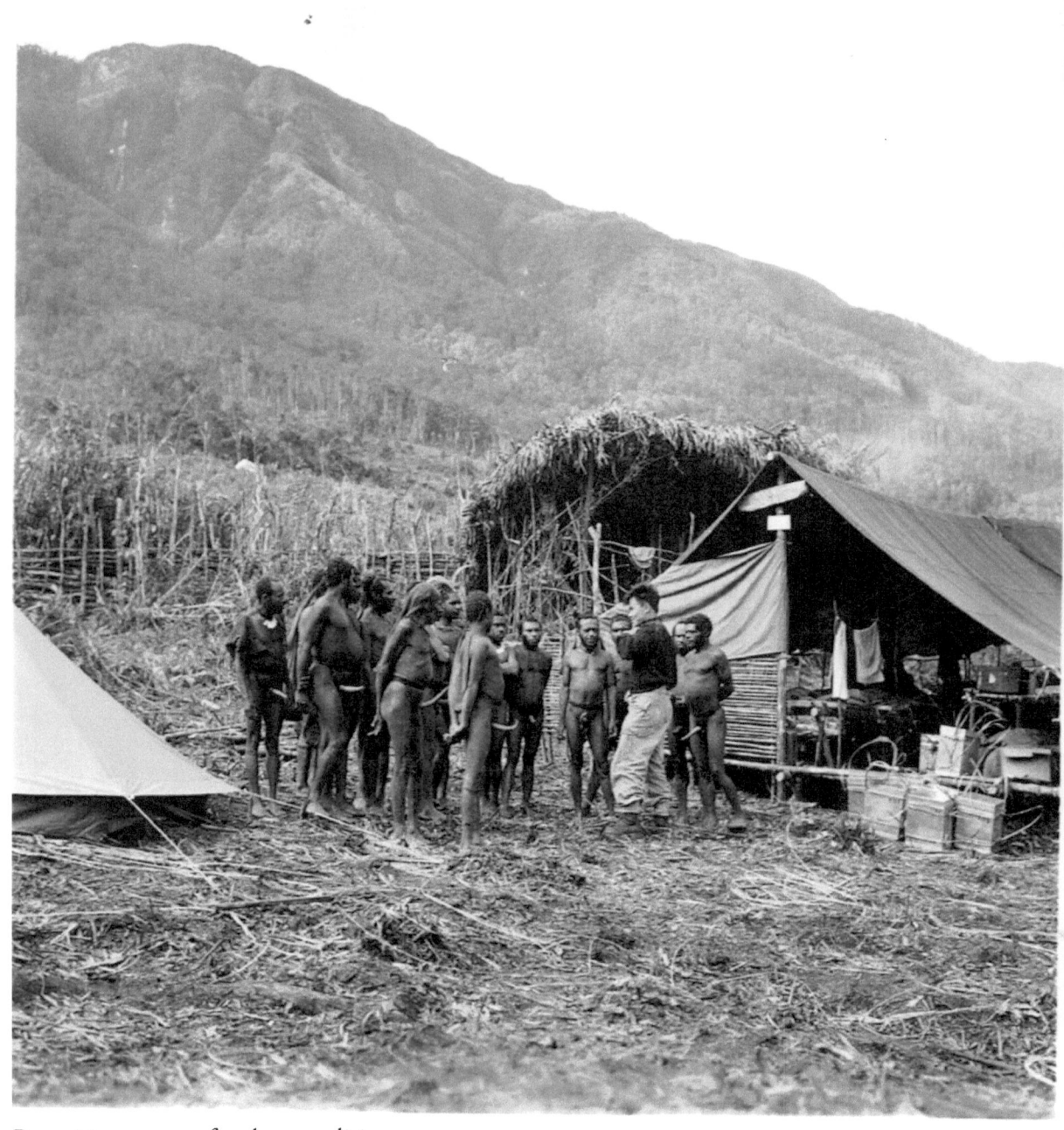

Recruiting porters for the expedition

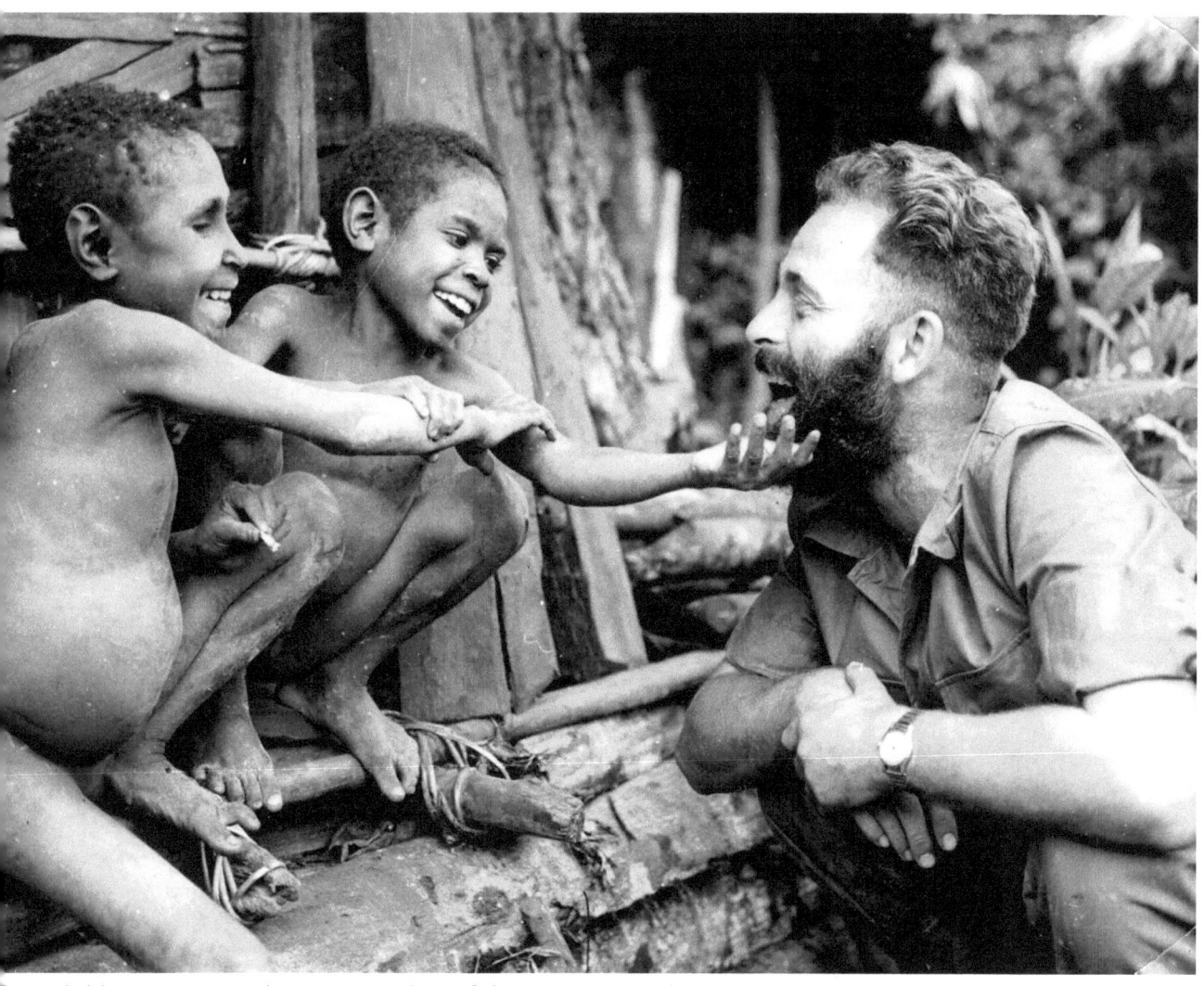

...age children getting to know a member of the Sterren expedition

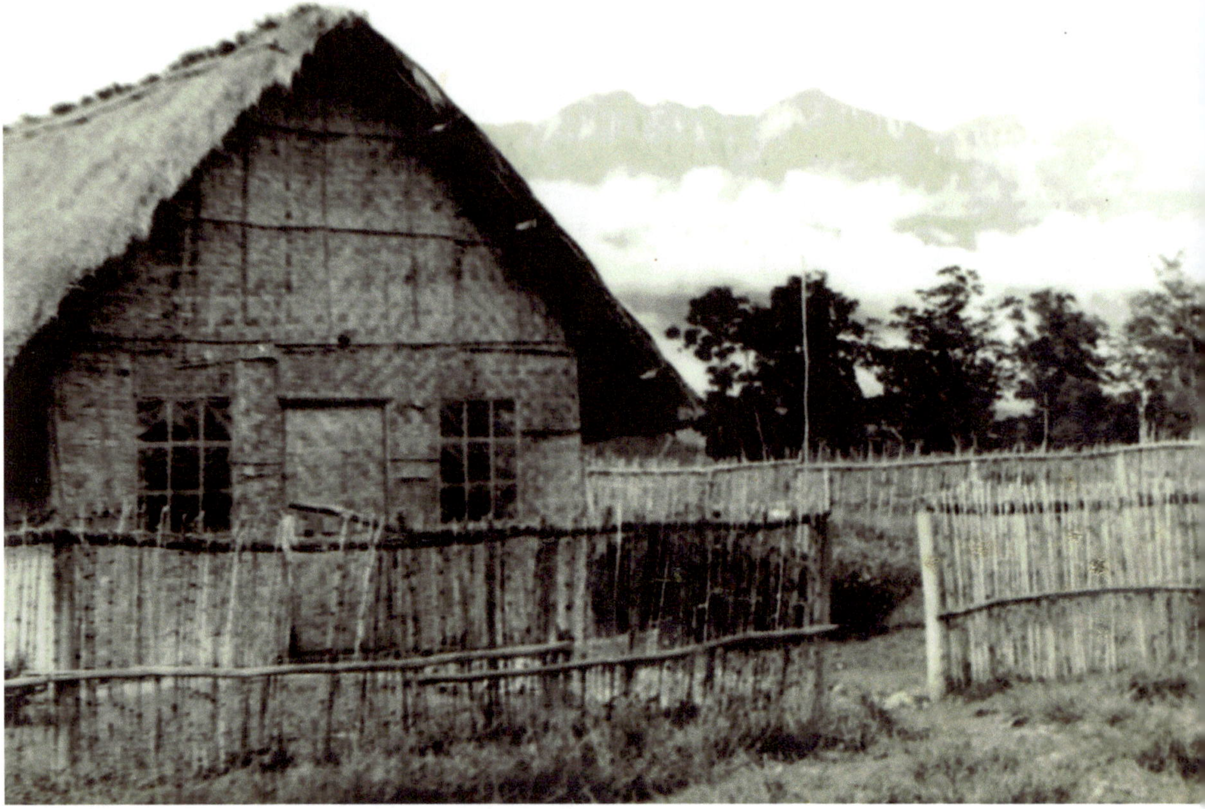

A home at the mission

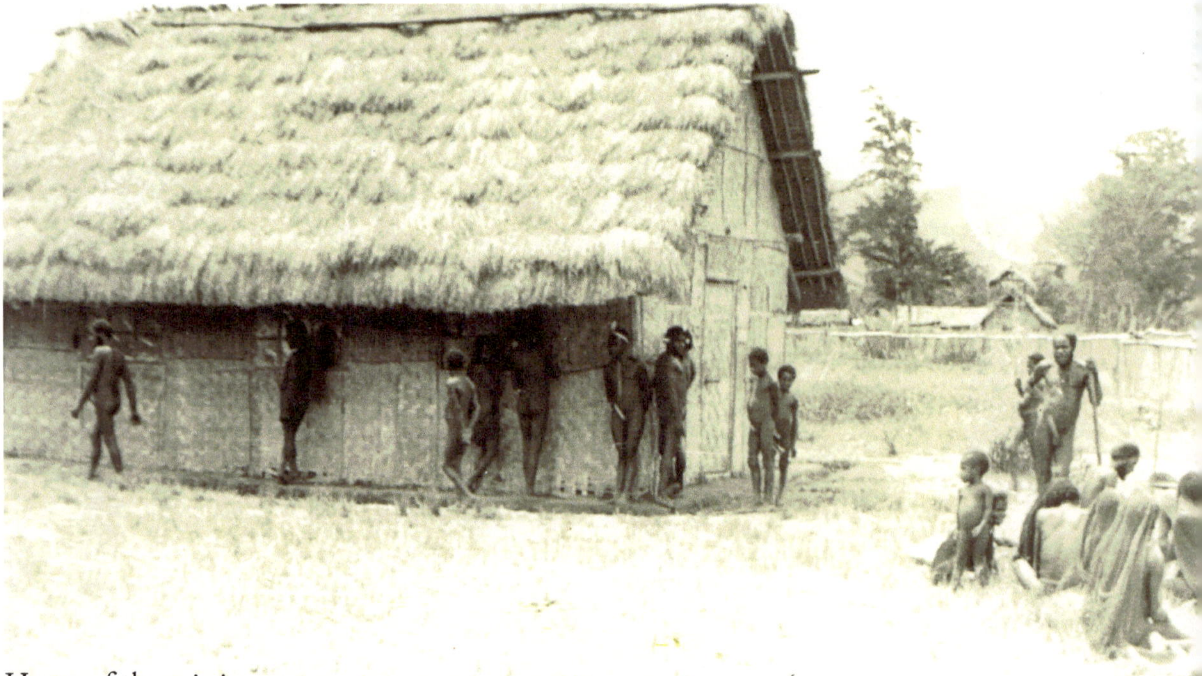

Home of the missionary

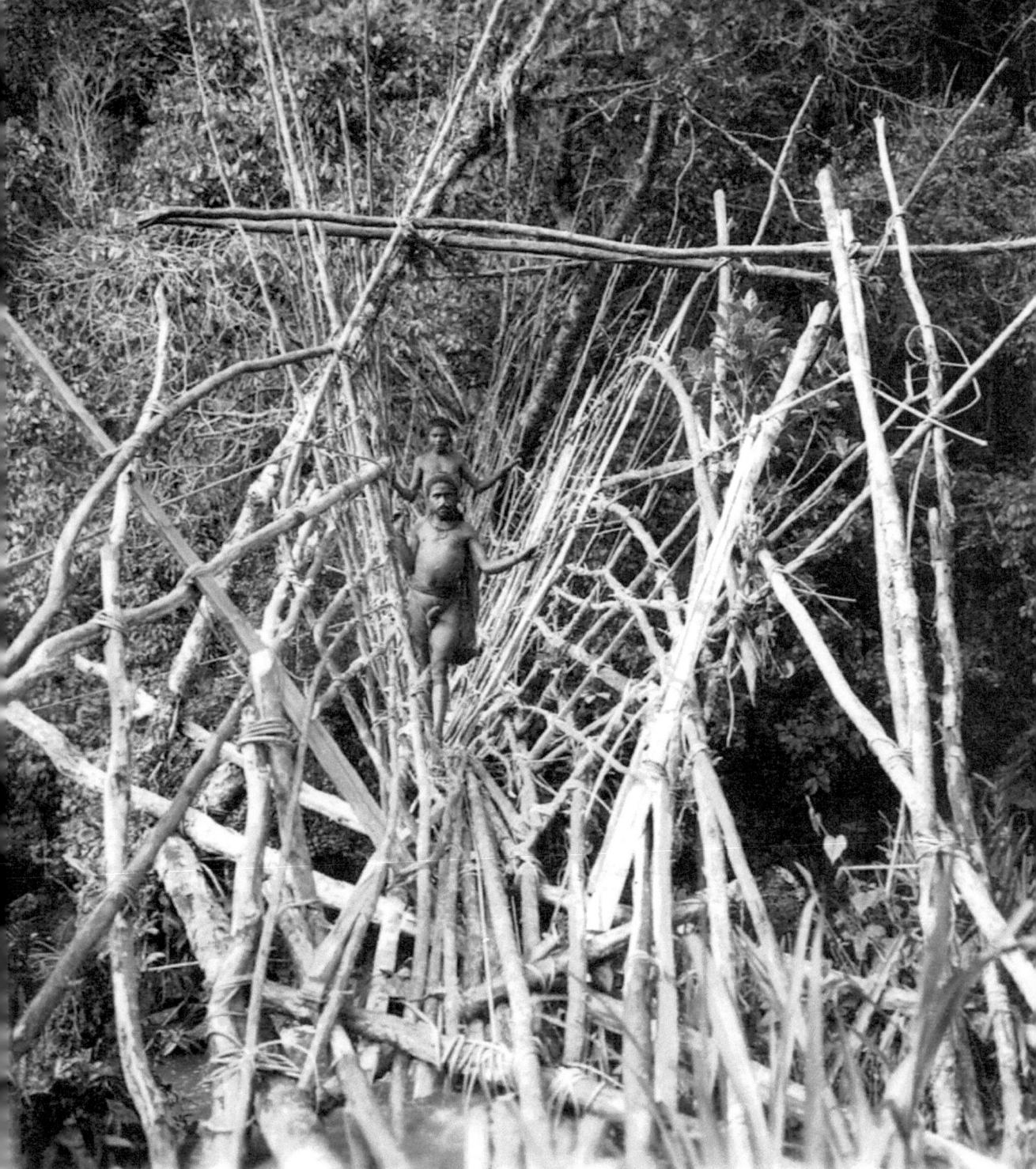

A bridge over a river in the Sterren Mountains

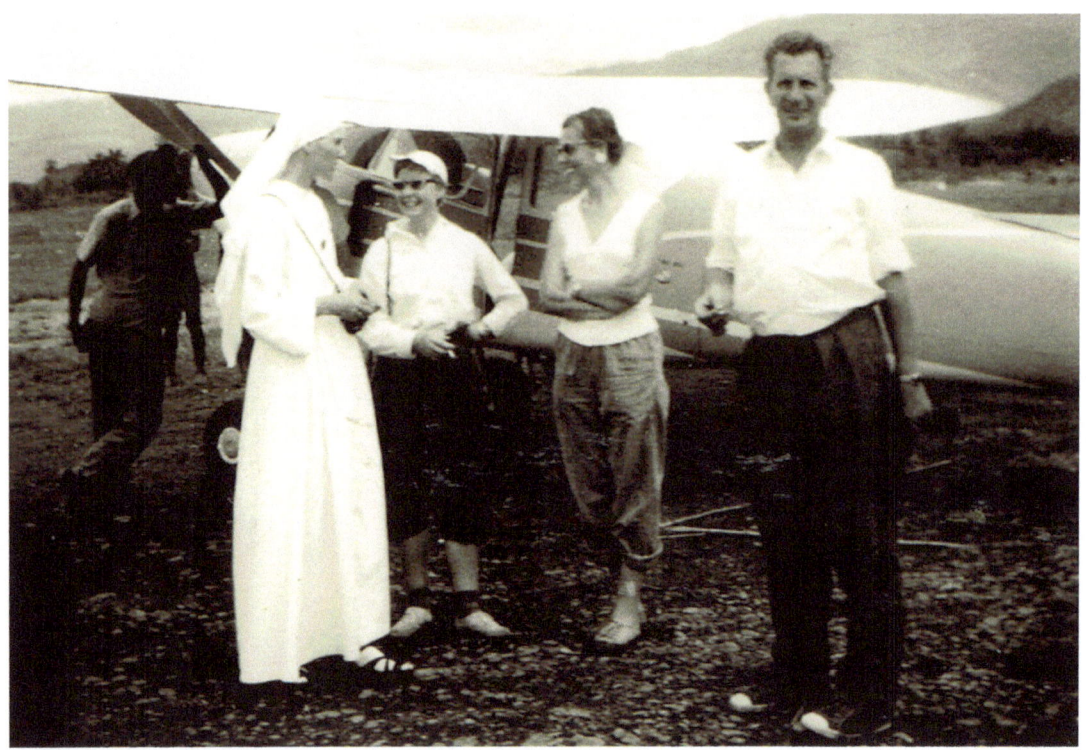
Arrival in Wissel Lake district, this sister is leaving with the Cessna

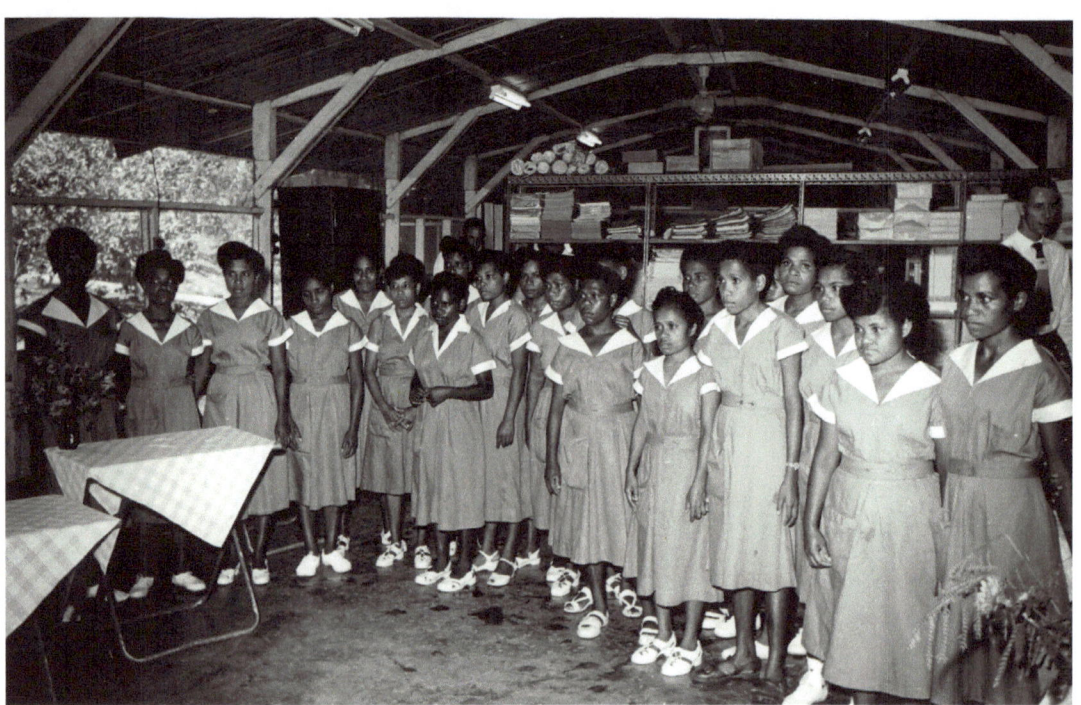
Health worker graduation

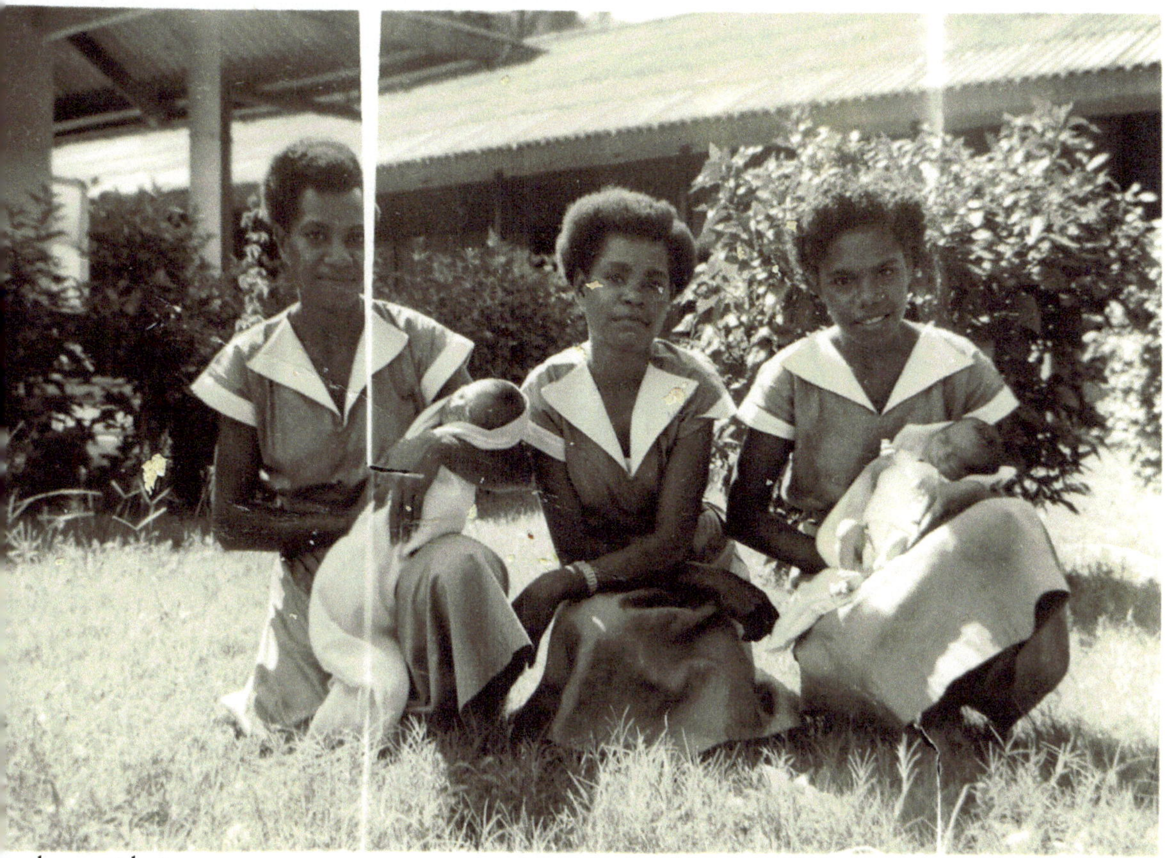

student midwives

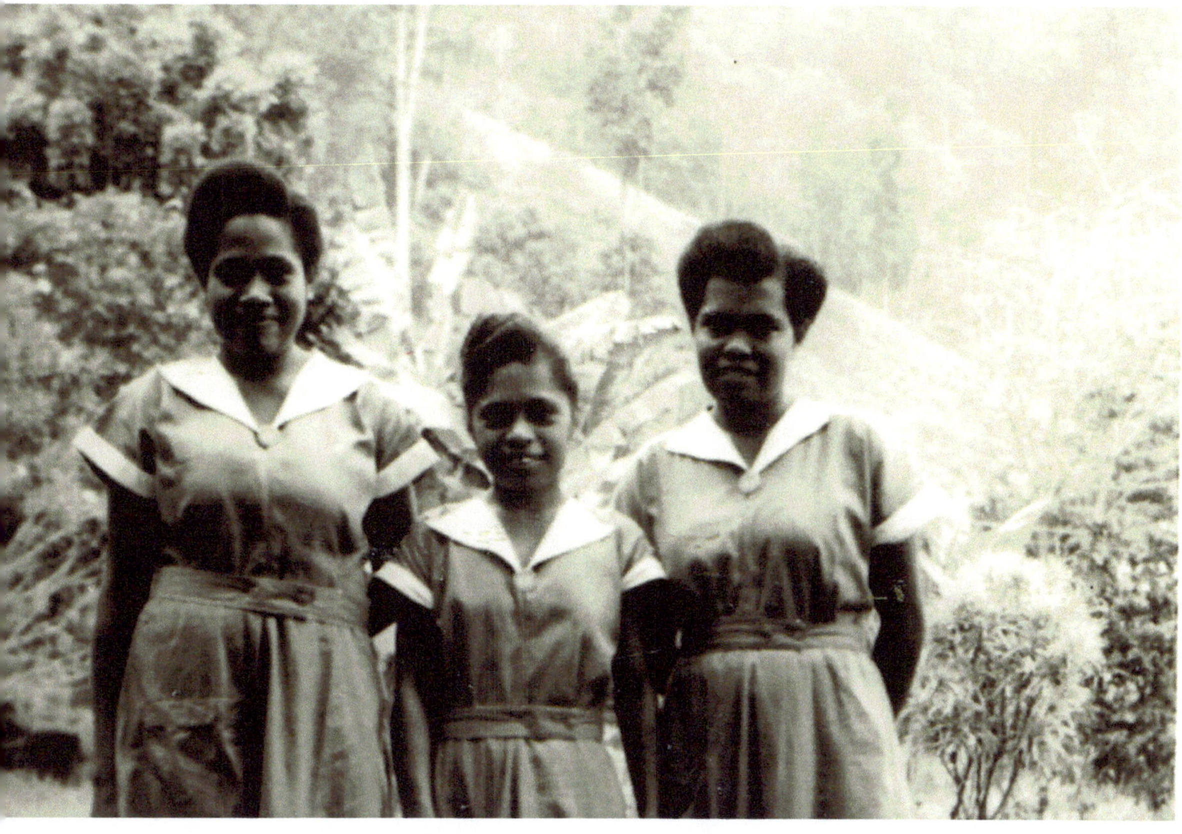

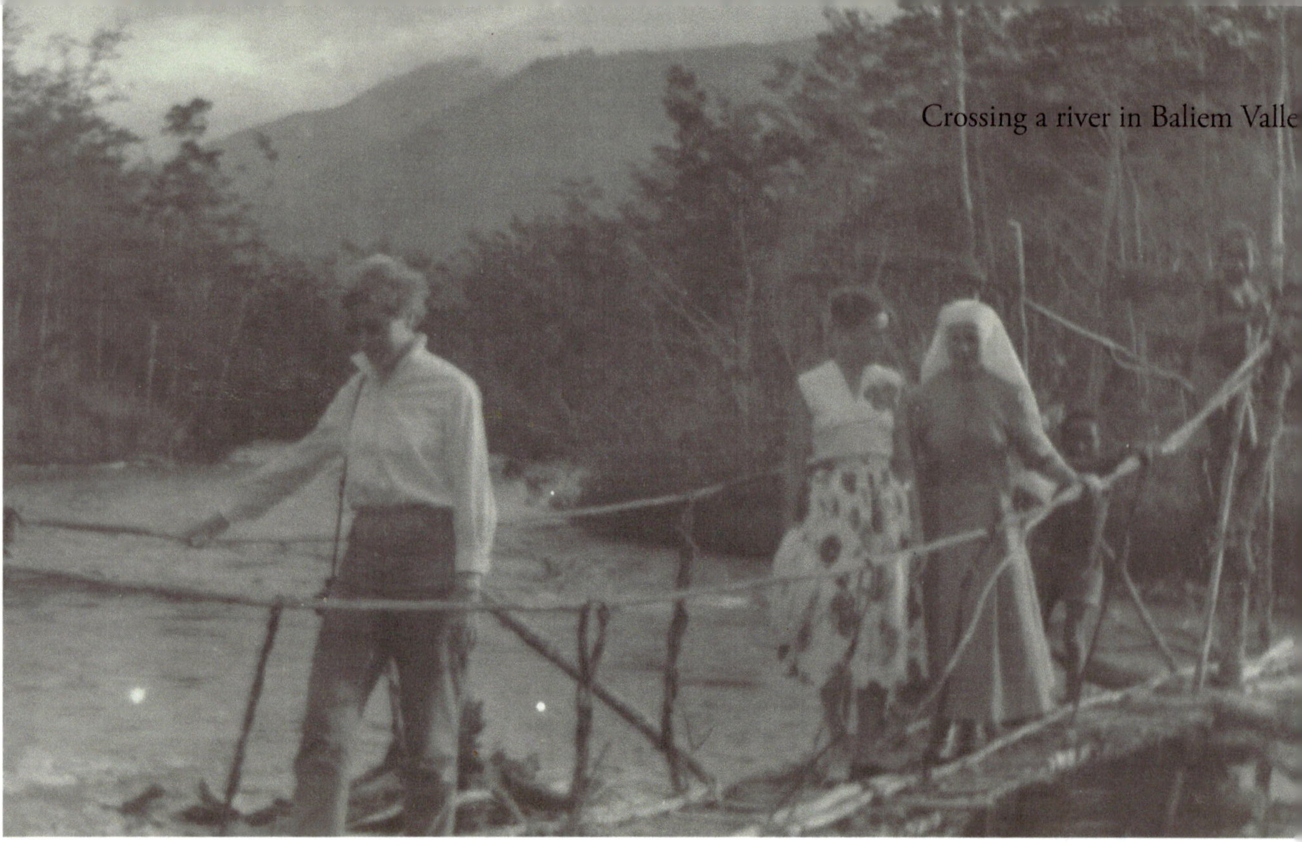

Crossing a river in Baliem Valley

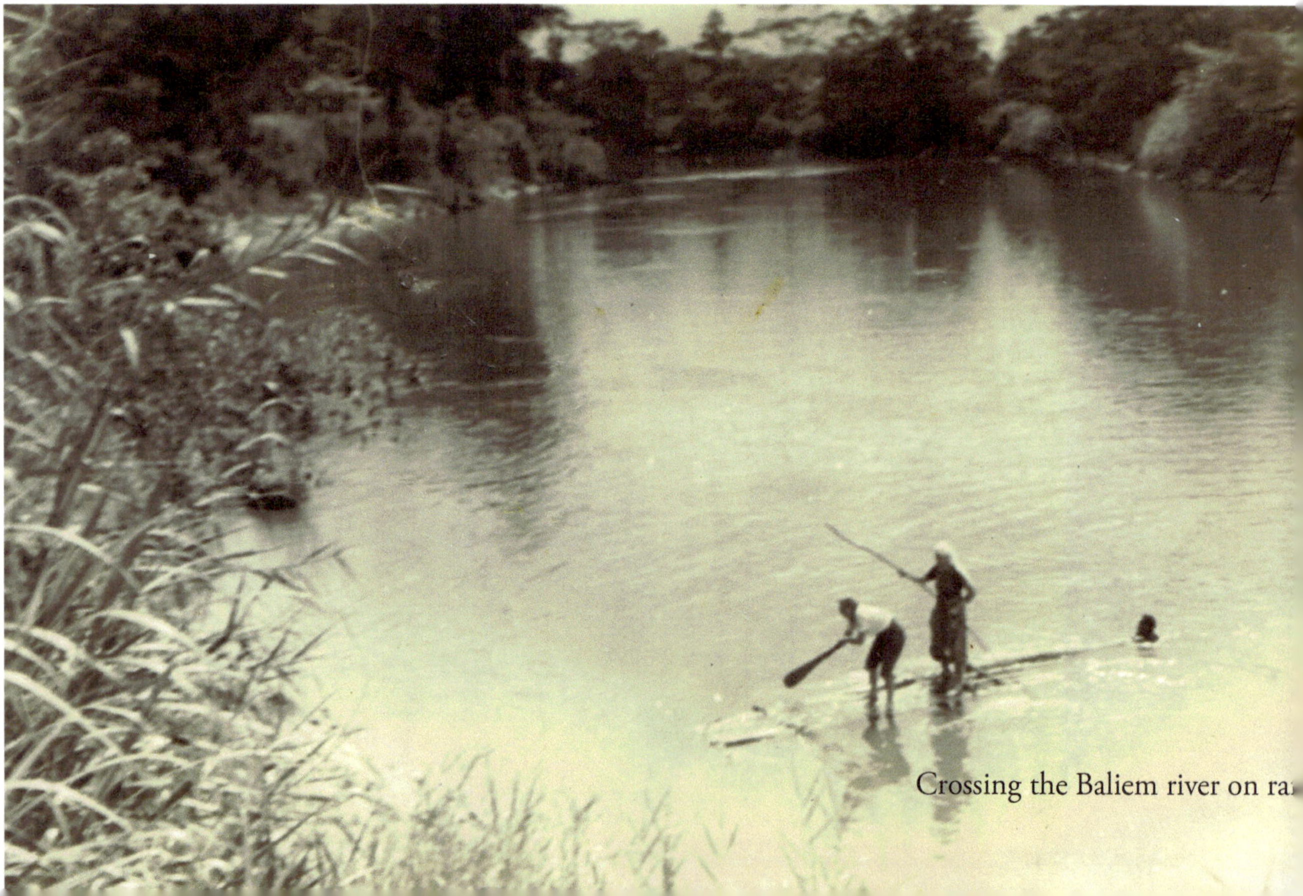

Crossing the Baliem river on raft

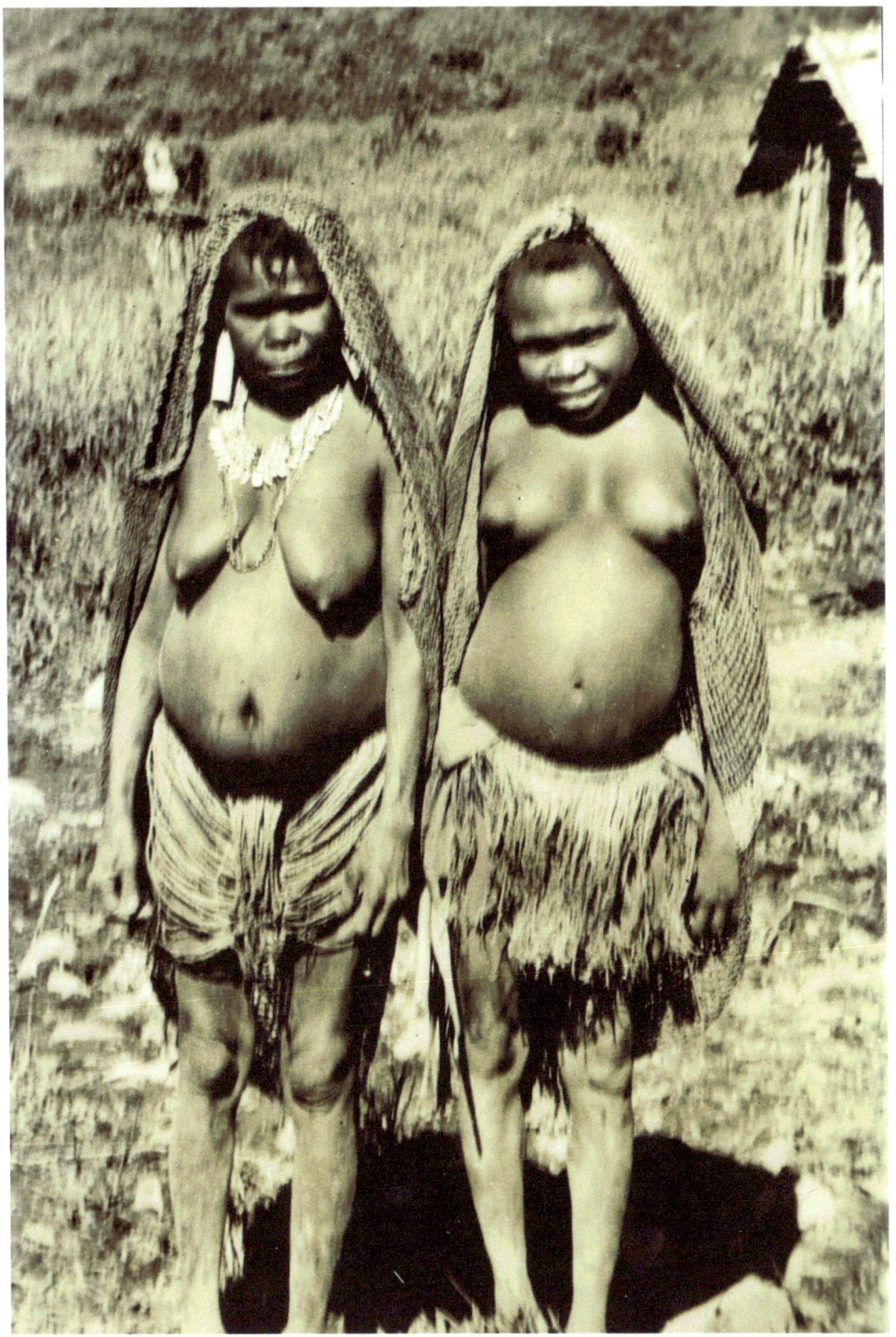

Married woman (left) and young girl (right), note the difference in grass skirts

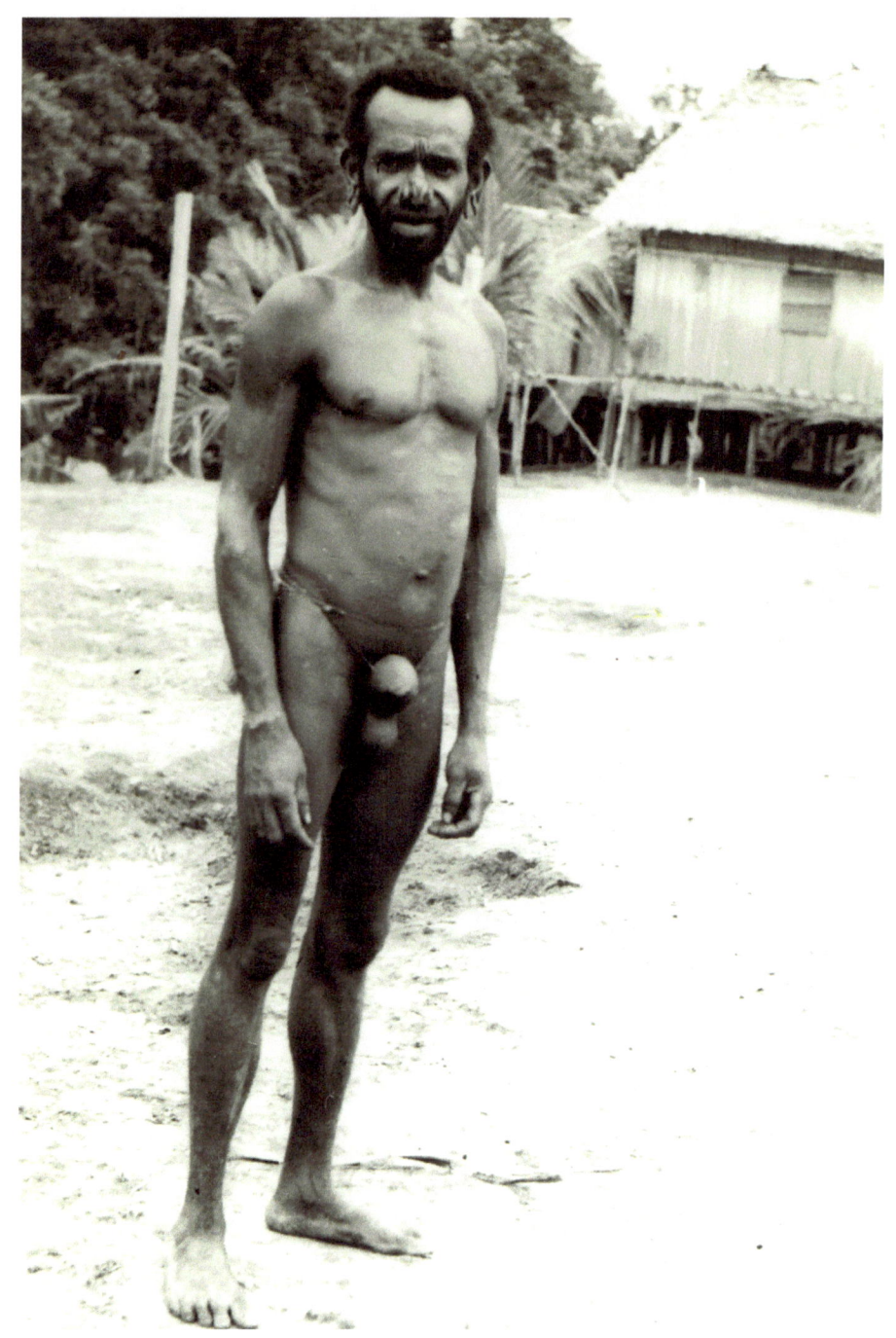

A man wearing typical clothing of just a shell

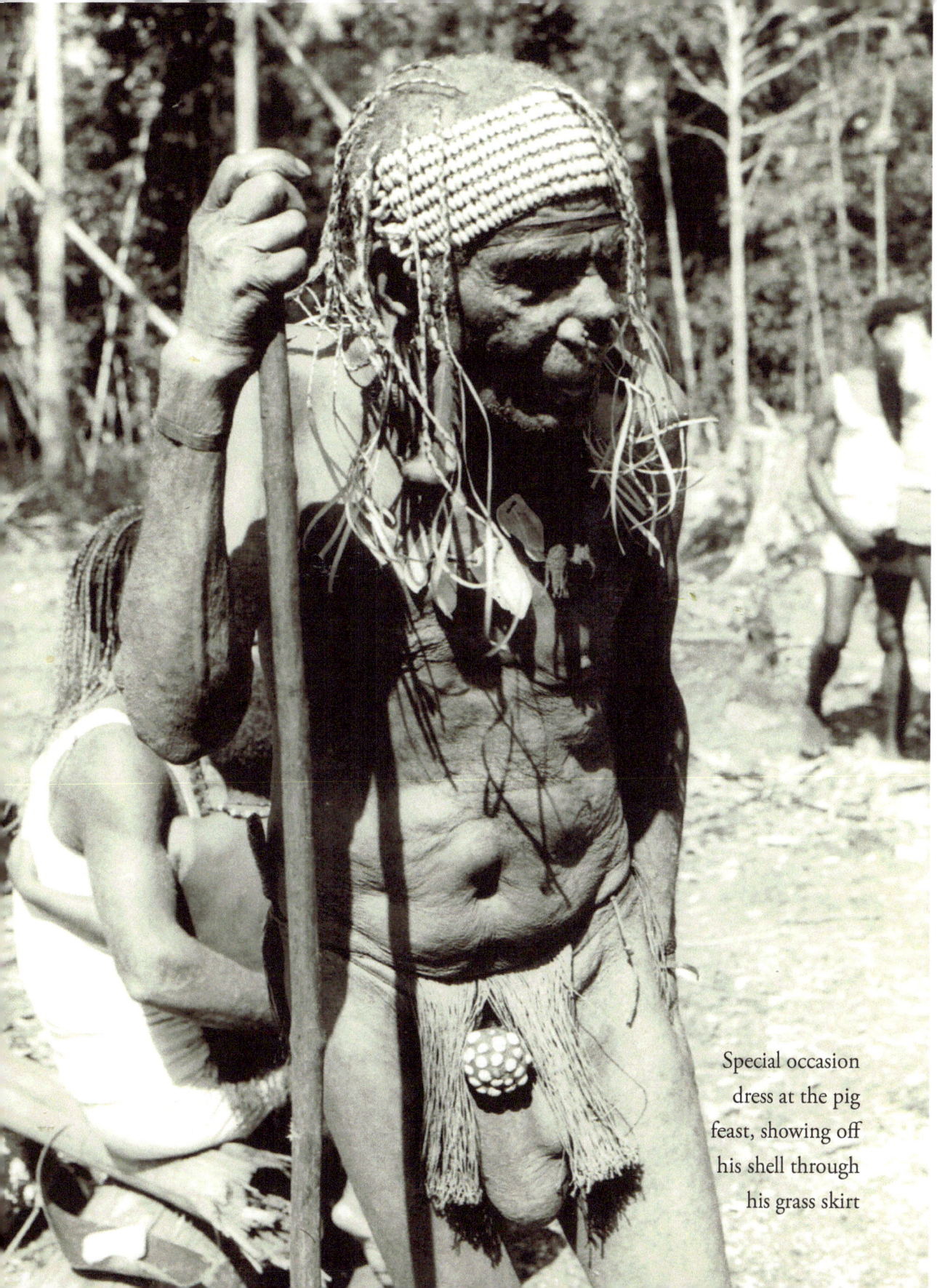

Special occasion dress at the pig feast, showing off his shell through his grass skirt

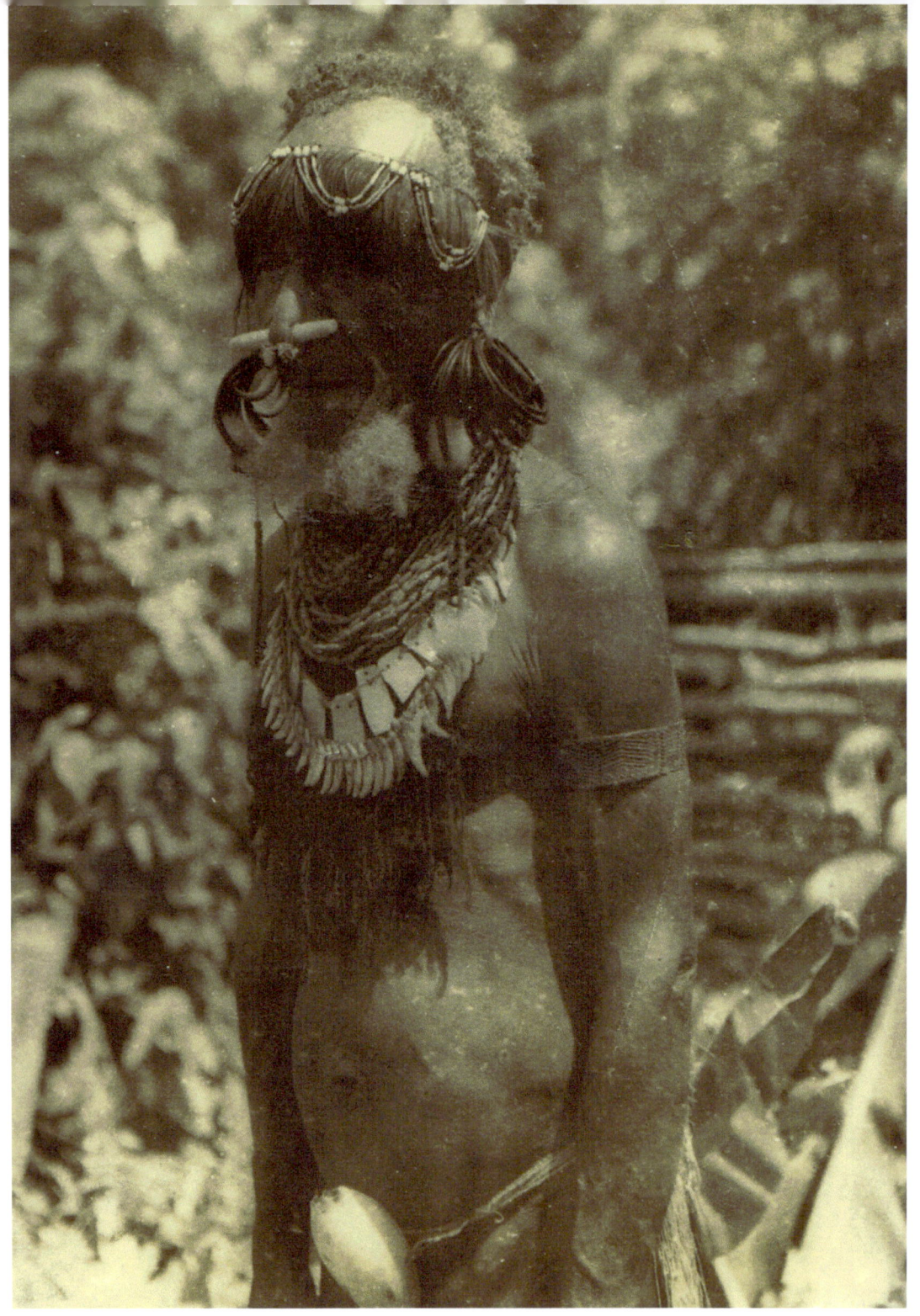

Note the pierced nose (piece of wood), earrings, headdress of bird feathers and string, he has a dufferent shell and a very ornate necklace made of pig and oxe teeth

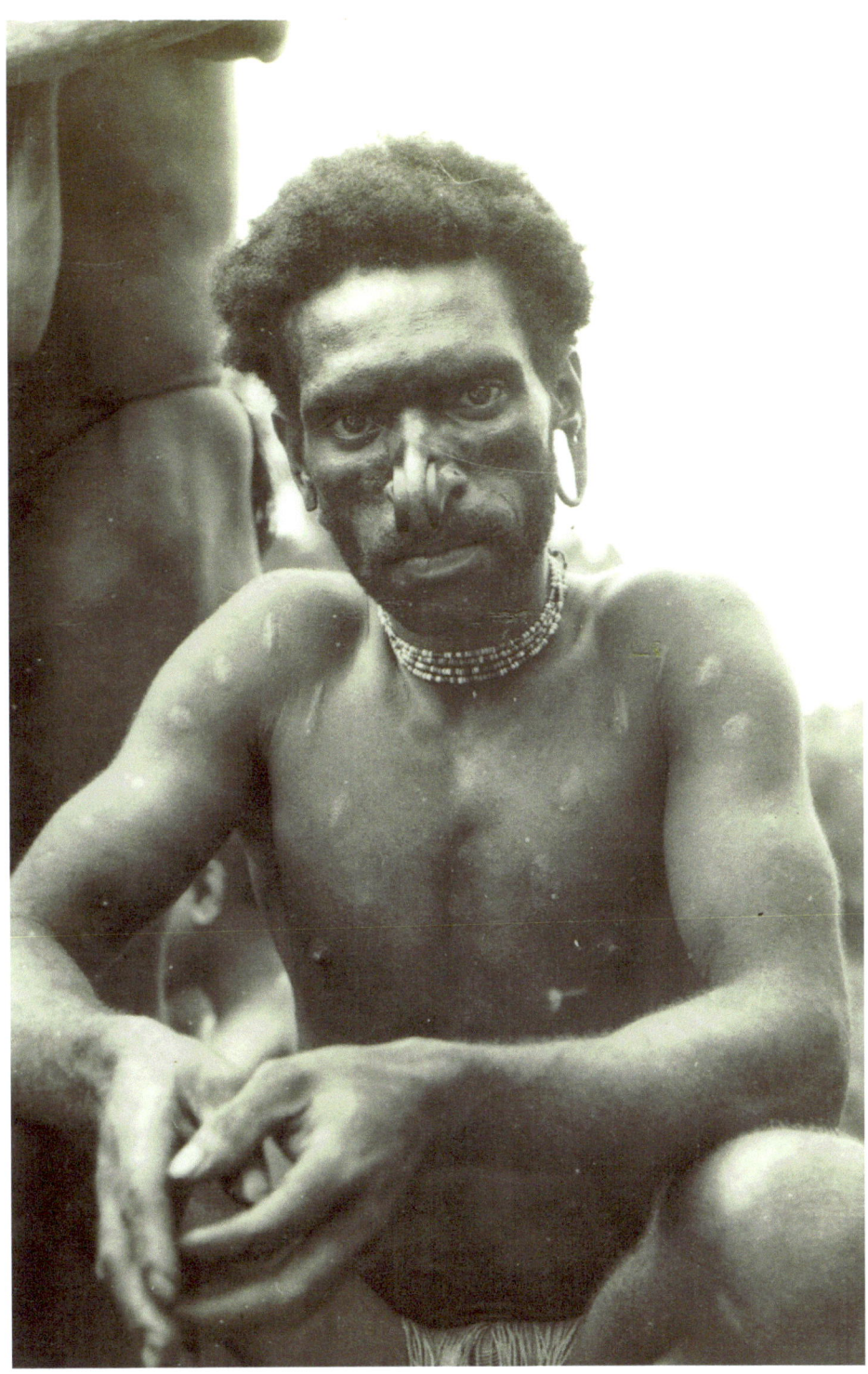
Note the stretched earlobe, 'my nose is pierced and decorated too'

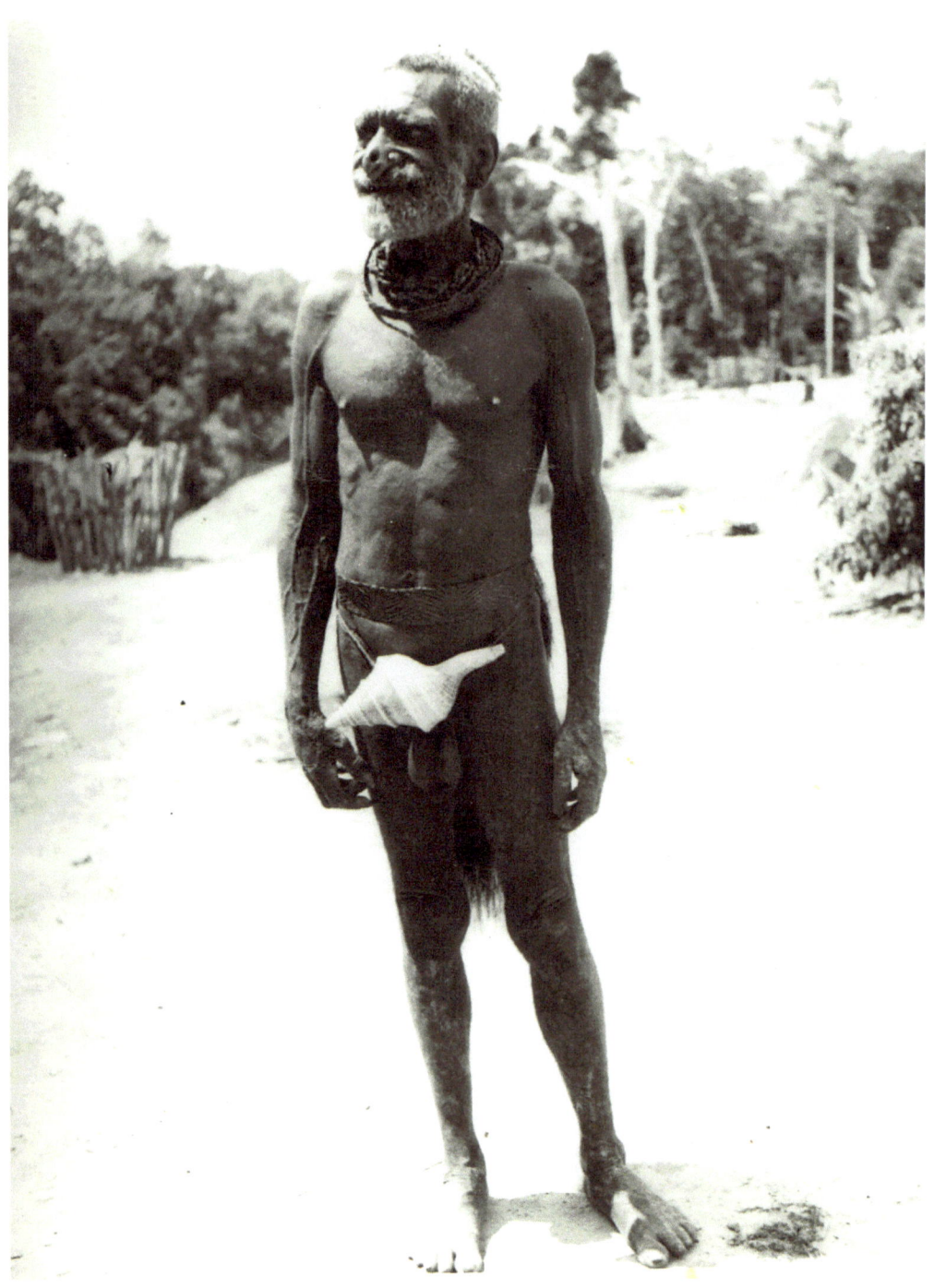

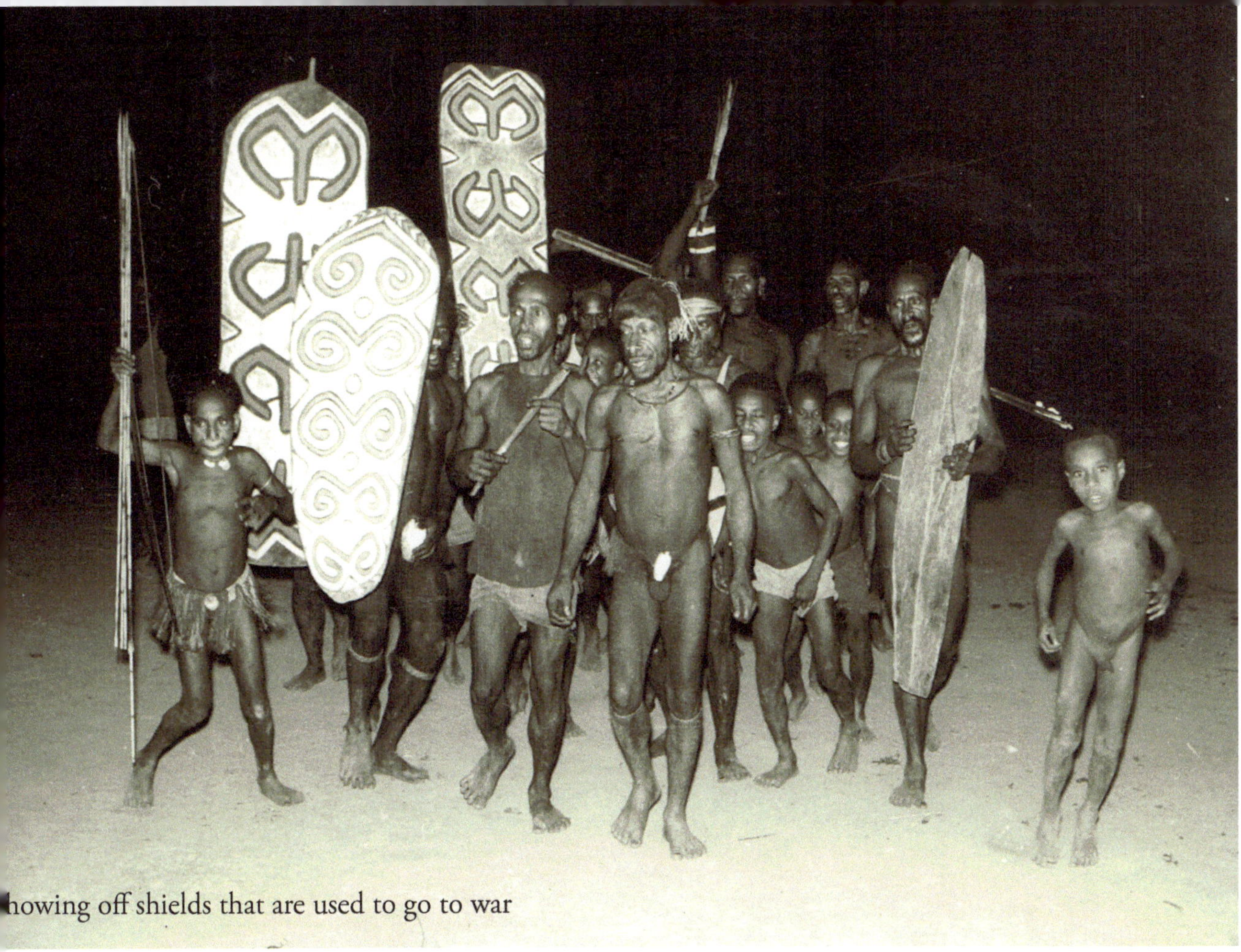

...howing off shields that are used to go to war

...960, The village's lookout tower in Baliem valley

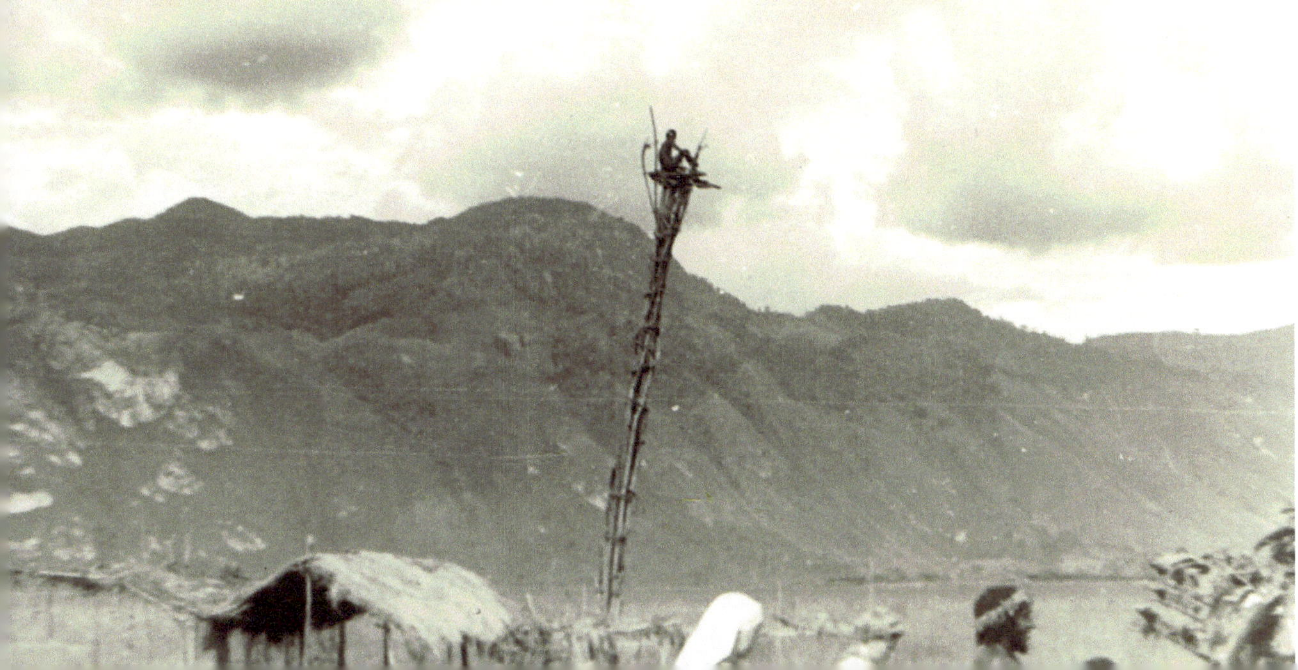

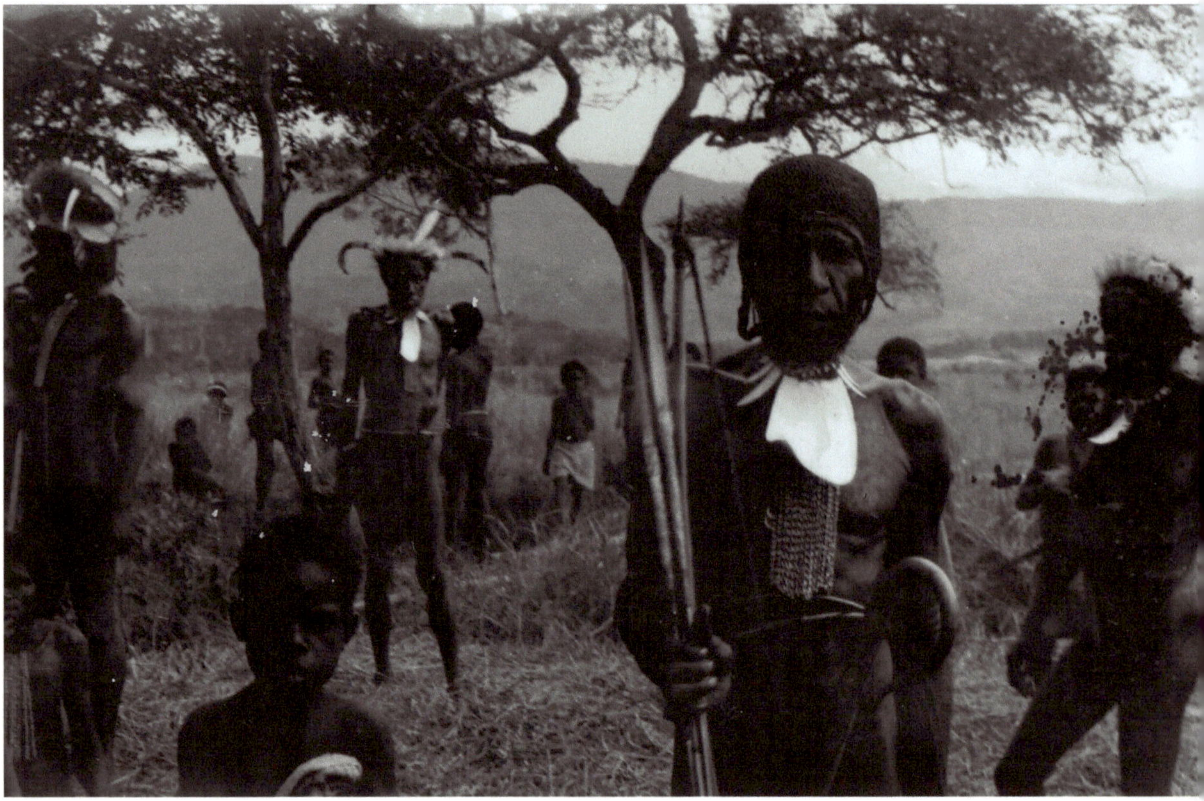

This man wears a gourd on his penis, Baliem Valley

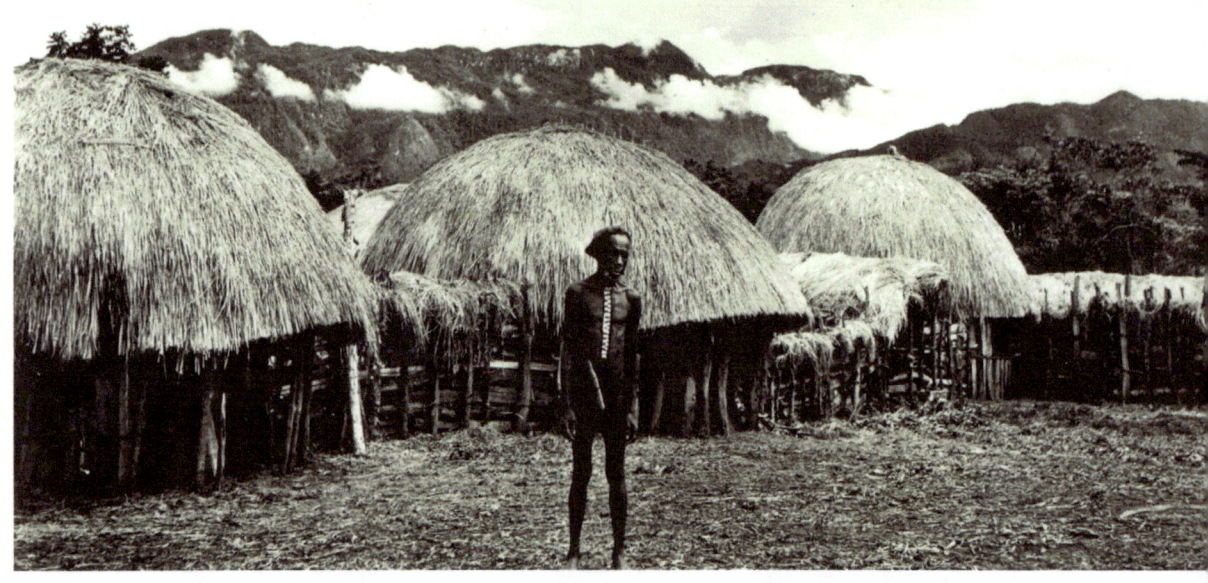

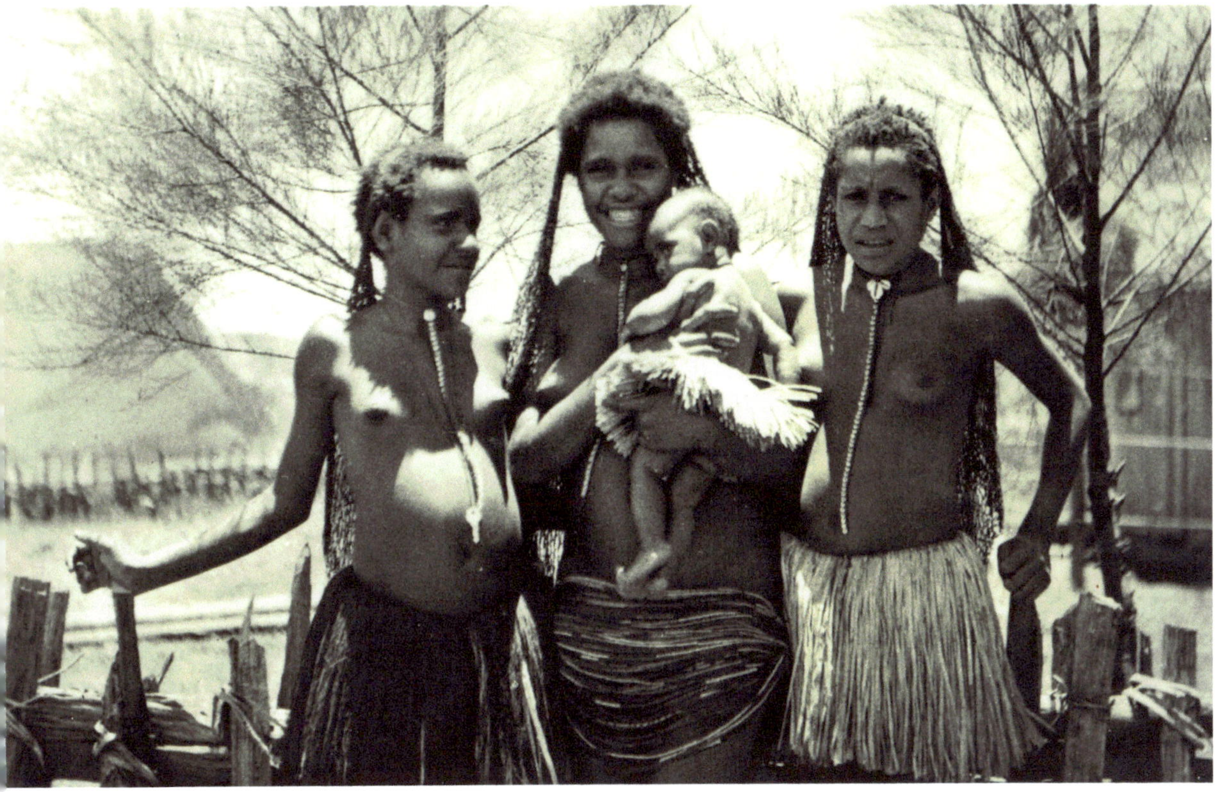

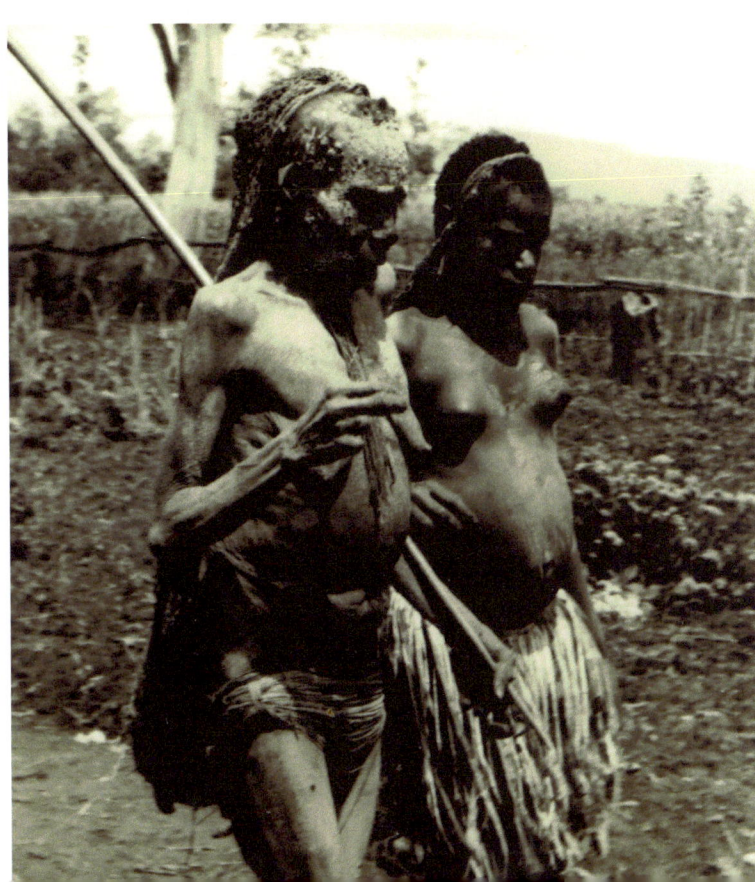

Old grandmother with her granddaughter

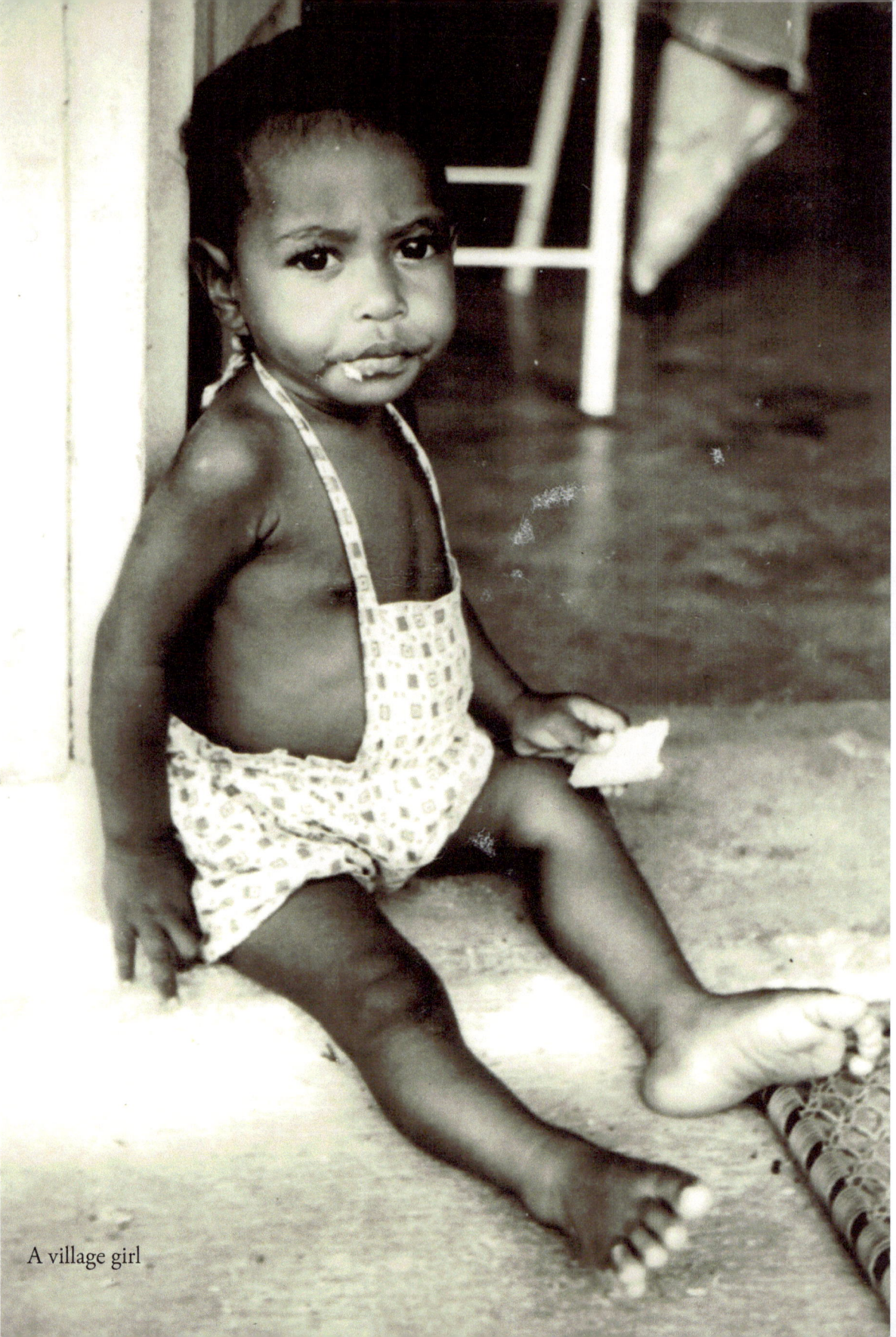
A village girl

RETURN TO HOLLAND

We left Hollandia by ship for Singapore. Ida had a friend whose aunt lived there, who had agreed that we could stay with her for a week. The aunt was married to an Indian lawyer and lived in a beautiful home and drove a jacquard in which she showed us all around Singapore.

It seemed unreal to us after living in such an undeveloped place for three and a half years. It was such a contrast! We had a ball! All the wonderful shops! And everywhere we went there was air conditioning! It was so cool everywhere! After a beautiful week, we boarded another ship to take us to Hong Kong where we spent another fabulous week.

From Hong Kong, we boarded the Nederwaal, a Dutch freighter with passenger accommodation for ten passengers. However, there were only four passengers. One couple and Ida and myself.

We were invited to eat at the captain's table for all our meals and told we could move freely on the ship and visit the bridge and engine room and crews lounge whenever we wanted.

It would be a six weeks journey to Amsterdam, and we would leave the

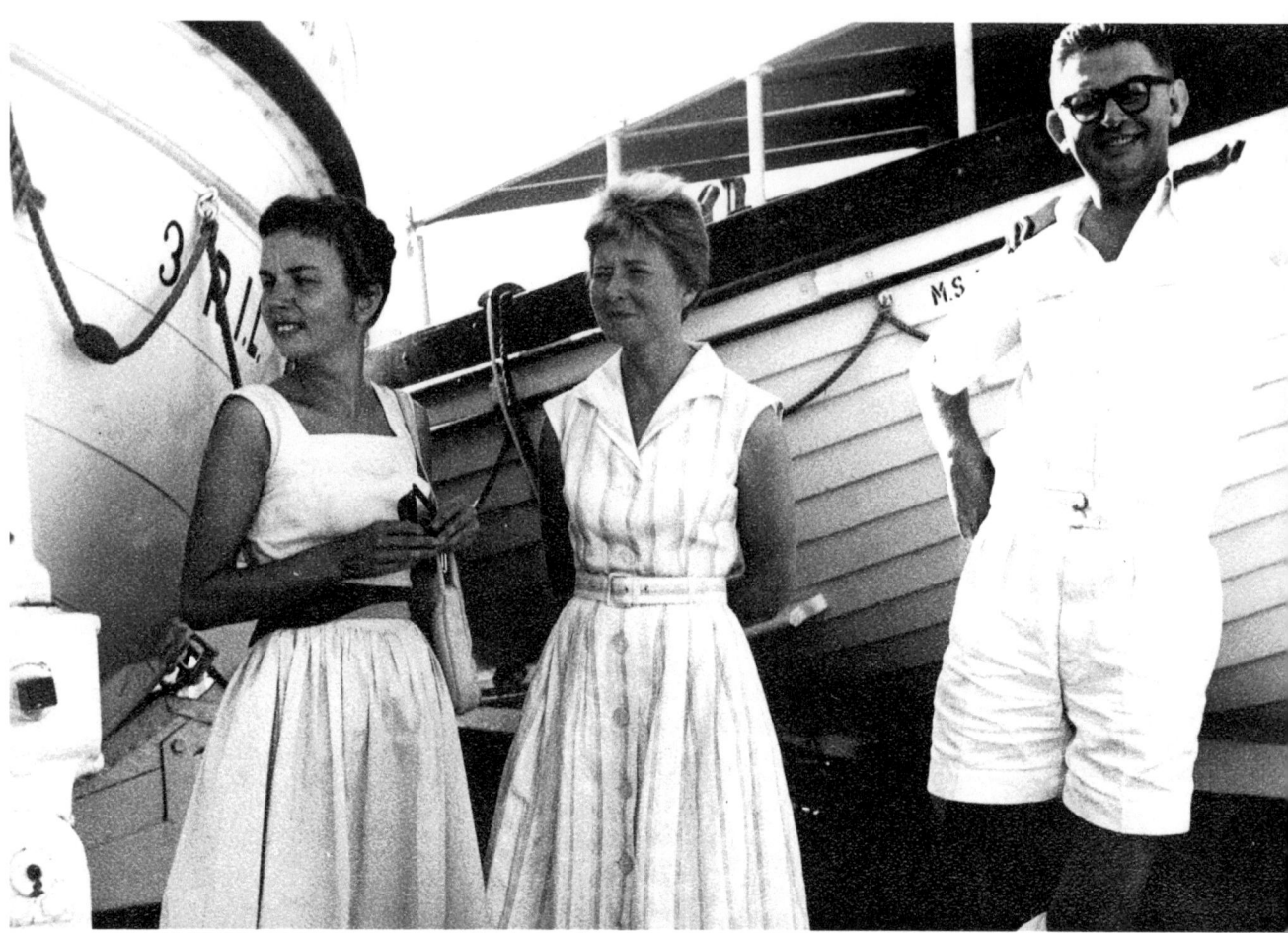

October 1961, on board the Nederwaal with Ida and a crew member

ship to 'do' Egypt over land. We had thought by camel, but that proved to be impossible. But, we did have a little ride on a camel at the pyramids in Cairo.

As the ship was a freighter, we had to make our own entertainment. We used our time to read a lot and write letters, which we posted in the various ports. We played pool with the crew, and one day we helped the crew painting the ship. We painted the boulders, white with red dots to make them look like mushrooms and had a good laugh. The captain pretended to be furious, but he most likely enjoyed the joke.

When asked at breakfast how we would like our eggs, we sometimes asked for them raw, much to the puzzlement of the waiter. Our hair and skin had suffered a fair bit from the sun at a time when sunscreen was not used in those days, so we pampered ourselves with egg face masks, and raw eggs are good for hair too.

The few days travelling through Egypt were exciting and Cairo was great, especially the museum. We would have liked to spend more time but had to rejoin our ship in Port Said. After Port Said, we stopped again in Alexandria, where we could get off and have a look around. What a beautiful city!

Next stop was Aden at the strait of Gibraltar, where I lost my watch. That is all I remember of Aden. Very busy and full of very pushy Arab shopkeepers. I had taken my watch off to wash my hand at a toilet, and when I realised and went back after only a minute, the watch was gone!

Oh well, I was very good at guessing the time, so I did not need a watch. From Aden, it was non-stop to Hamburg first and then to Amsterdam.

Of course, I had written home to let the family know when the ship was arriving. I remember standing at the railing looking at the people on the quay when Ida asked me, "are those people there your family? They are waving at us" I very stupidly said, "no, my mother does not have a broken arm". But it was

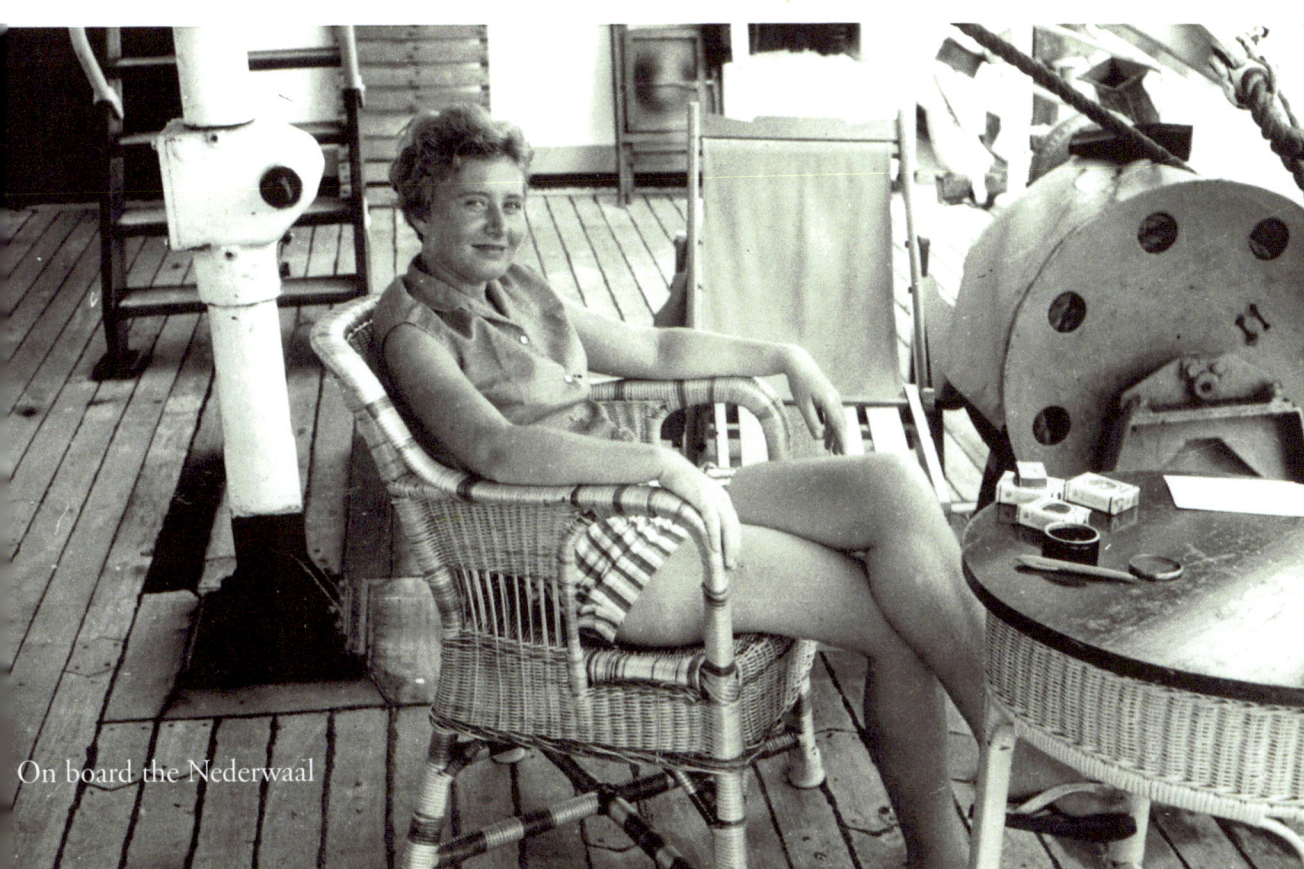

On board the Nederwaal

my family!! My mother had that very morning broken her wrist falling over a pair of shoes. She was rushed to the doctor and told him to hurry up as she was meeting her daughter. And she made it on time!

We often laughed about it later on how I had said, "no that is not my family, my mother does not have a broken arm". How could I possibly have known? What a blessing that I was home now, as I could take care of mum and run the household, as mum could not do a thing with one arm.

I noticed that mum was quite overweight again and asked her if she would like to lose some weight. She said yes, and as I was preparing the meals anyway, this worked wonderfully. She lost thirty kilograms over the next few months, and although she often told me that she felt like a rabbit, giving her so many raw vegetables, she was pleased as she did never feel hungry and was happy to lose the weight.

This is the only time that my mum was not overweight apart from the wartime. She always had such a healthy appetite, and did it really matter? She did live to ninety-nine! She was always active and healthy and walked everywhere as long as she could. I probably just wanted to prove a point, being a nurse.

By now mum had fully recovered, and I was getting restless. During this time, I did a bit of part-time work in a new hospital in Buitenveldert. Ida's parents lived there too, so we stayed in touch while deciding what to do next.

As we both had been working as midwives in NG but were not qualified midwives, we thought it might be a good idea to do our training. In Holland, it takes two years, but in Britain, you can do it in one year. We found a hospital in Edinburg Scotland, prepared to take us on as student midwives. The training is divided into two parts. Part one is in the hospital and part two in the district. In each part one has to do twenty deliveries under supervision, each part taking six months.

SCOTLAND AND LONDON

Doing a postgraduate course in a foreign language was a challenge. We both had studied English in high school some ten years ago and had never learnt any medical terminology.

Ida found it a lot harder than I did, which puzzled our colleagues. I seem to have more natural ability for languages. Ida worked a lot harder on the theory. The fact that we had done a six-month maternity training after our general did help. Also, our years of experience in NG was a great help. We had no problem with the practice of delivering babies.

One particular sister in charge used to get quite frustrated with me, not always understanding her strong Scottish accent, after reporting on each patient in the morning, I would sometimes ask, "sister, what about Mrs Jones?" She would shout, "Nurse Blommesteyn, I have just told you!"

And I would answer, "yes that may be so, but I did not get it, could you please repeat it?" As I was supposed to look after that patient for the day, I felt I needed to know the details.

We were lucky that we did our training at the Elsie Inglis Hospital and not at the Royal Edinburgh, as we heard from some of the girls who did their training there that they had difficulty getting their twenty deliveries in, as that hospital also trained medical students.

I do remember two particular cases from my time at the Elsie Inglis. I once delivered a baby without arms. This was 1961 when the drug thalidomide was given during pregnancy for morning sickness. This drug, unbeknown at the time sometimes caused malformations in the baby, mainly missing limbs. The other case I remember was a baby I was concerned about. I just felt there was something wrong. I told the sister in charge, but she told me I imagined it. I decided to speak to the paediatrician, who took me seriously, did a thorough check and diagnosed a heart defect. The baby was operated upon, and the paediatrician came to thank me for bringing my concern to her attention.

It was during this time in Scotland that I met Adel Chaban, an Egyptian doctor who was studying in Edinburgh for his RFCS. I do not recall how we met, but it must have been at a party. We became very close, but the fact that he was a Muslim although not very strict and I was Catholic, also not very strict, remained a problem.

For the second half of our training, we had to go around the district on a bicycle, much like the current television series "Call The Midwife". We had to do twenty home deliveries and care for mother and baby at home.

The homes we visited had no heating, so we had to make a fire and bath the baby in front of the fire on our lap. Although most houses had a bathtub, this was mostly used to store coal or firewood, but seldom to bathe. Whether we worked in a particularly poor part of Edinburgh, I don't know, but I was quite surprised at how primitive most homes were.

Once I was given an address to care for a newborn and mother, and when I got there, there was a baby but no mother. I made a fire and bathed the baby and by this time still no mother. I decided I could not leave the baby although I had quite a few more patients to attend. After a few hours, my supervisor came to see what was keeping me. She agreed that I should not leave. The mother came home eventually saying, she just went down the road to see a friend! She was severely reprimanded by the supervisor. She was very young and could not understand that what she did was wrong.

Adel Chaban

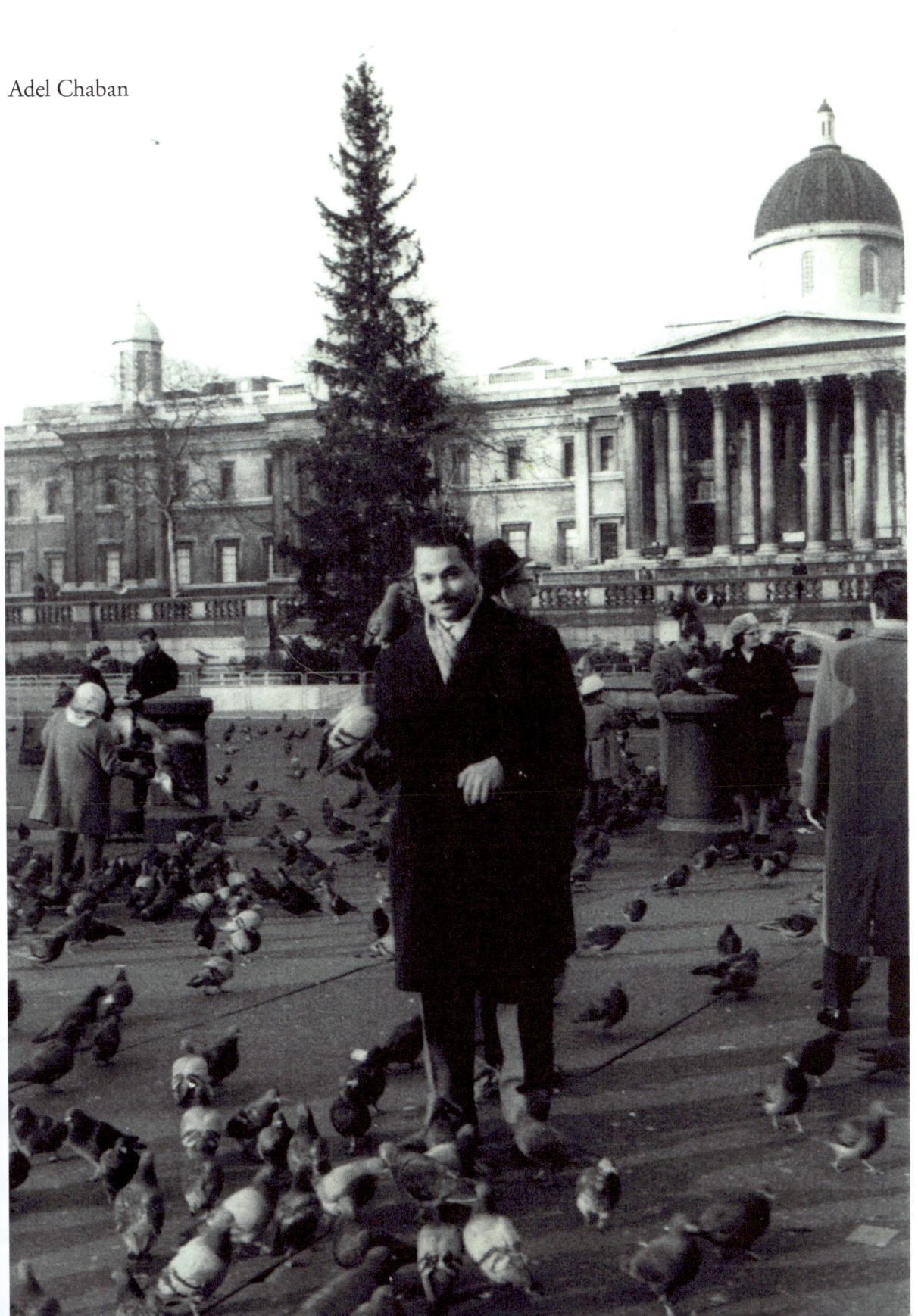

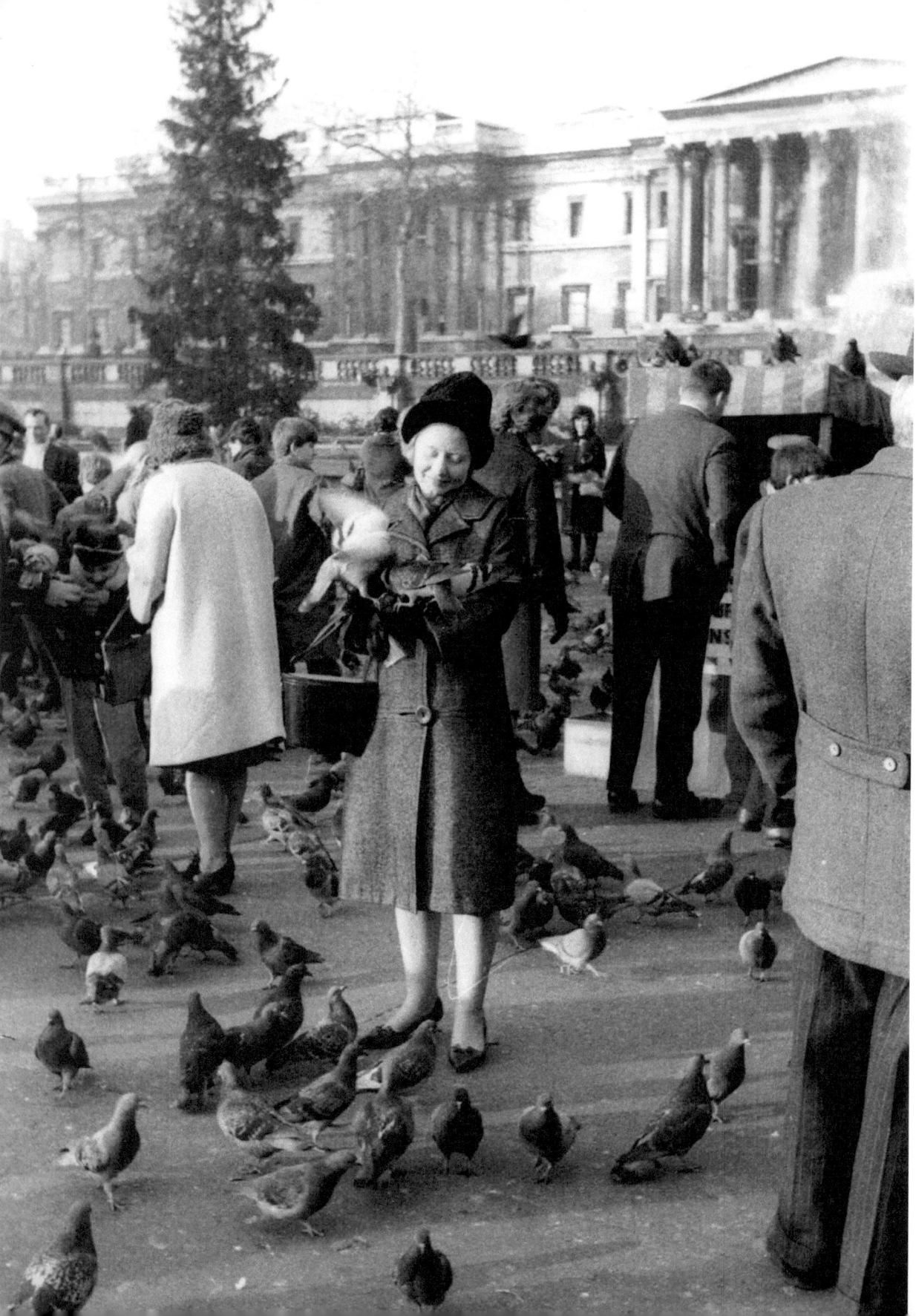

Ida and I both passed our exams and got our midwifery certificates. Ida went back to Holland. As Adel had finished his theoretical part and went to London for his practice as a surgeon, I decided to go to London and do a six month theatre training course at Camberwell Hospital. This was not far from the hospital where Adel was, so we kept seeing each other.

I enjoyed working in the theatre, and as I still had my Vespa scooter, I did see some of the surrounds on my days off. I often went to Brighton in summer. If the weather was not good, I visited some of the museums. London was not so busy then, and I was quite comfortable driving around on my scooter. On the rare occasion that Adel was off on the same day, we would spend the day sightseeing together.

After six months Adel went back to Egypt, and I went back to Amsterdam. We never saw or heard from each other again. I was heartbroken, but it would not have worked. I did love him very much and often wondered how his life turned out.

Did he still think about me?

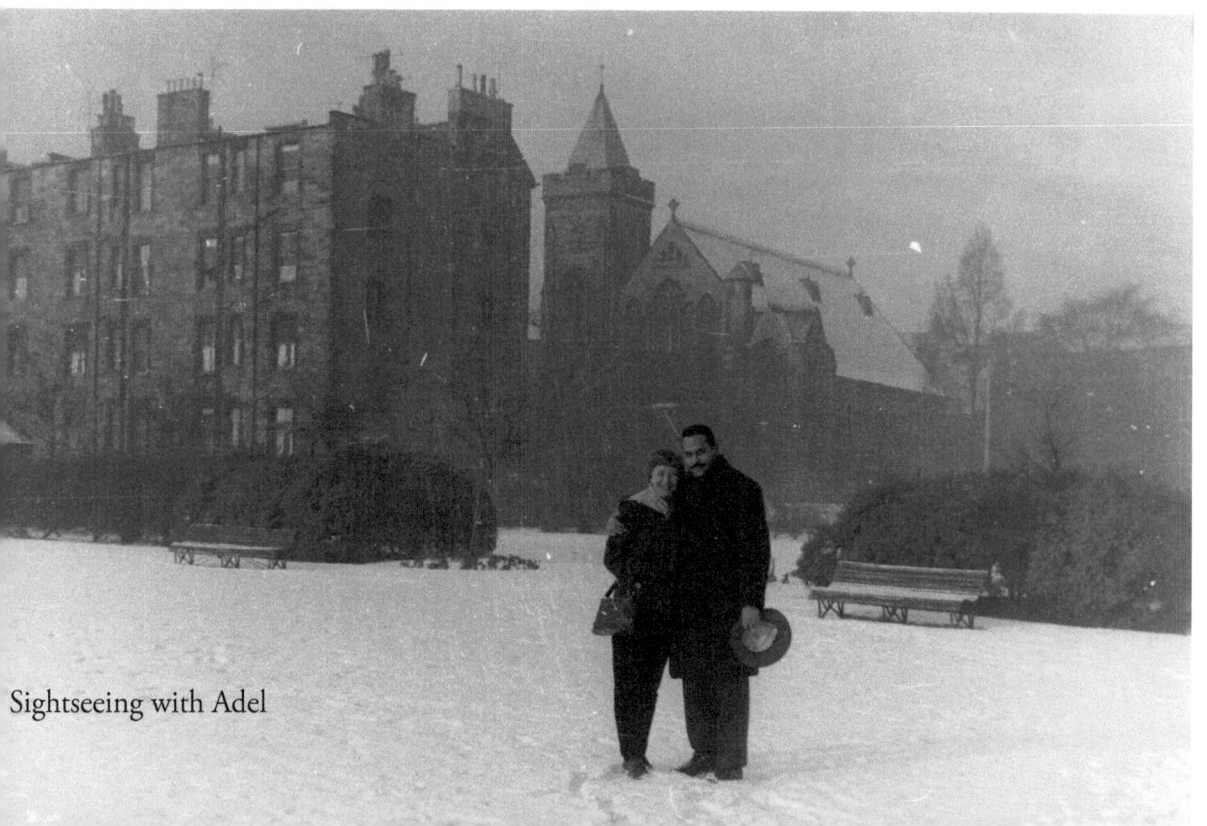

Sightseeing with Adel

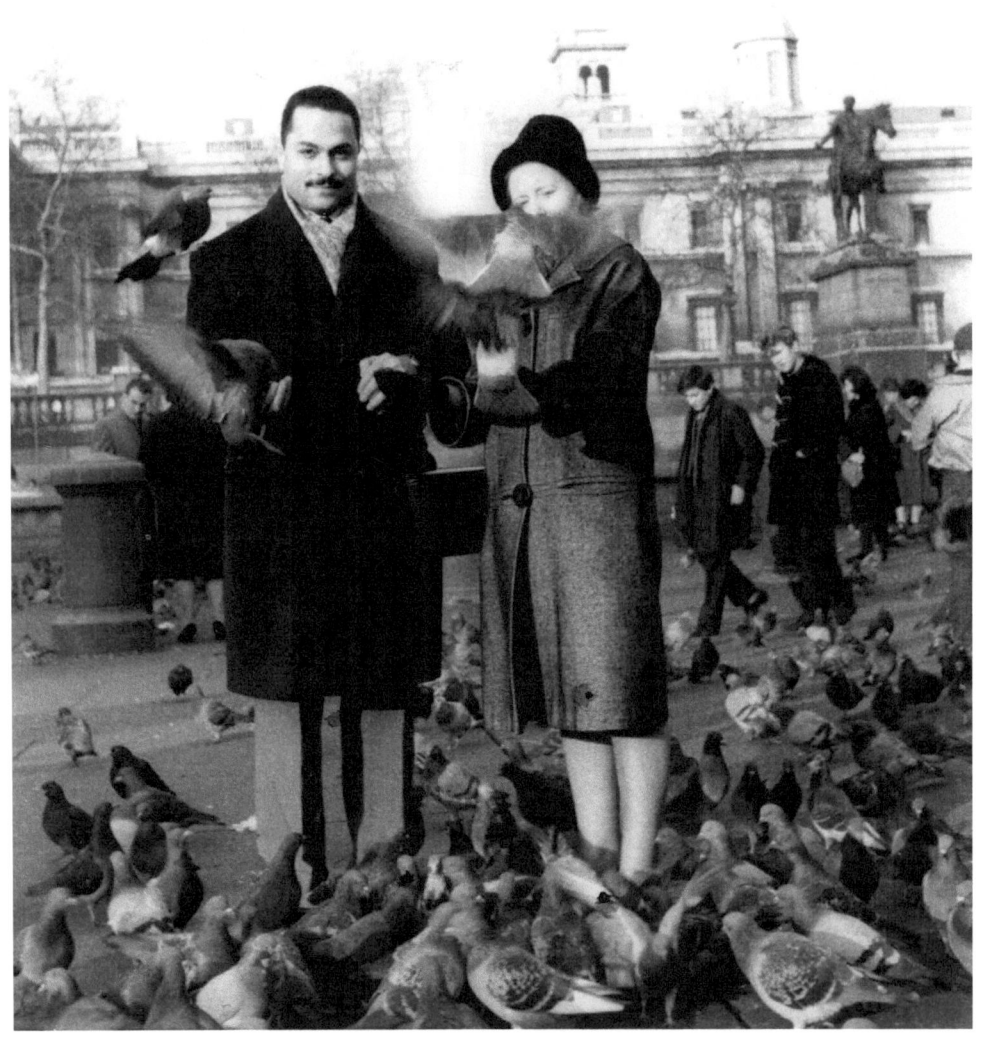

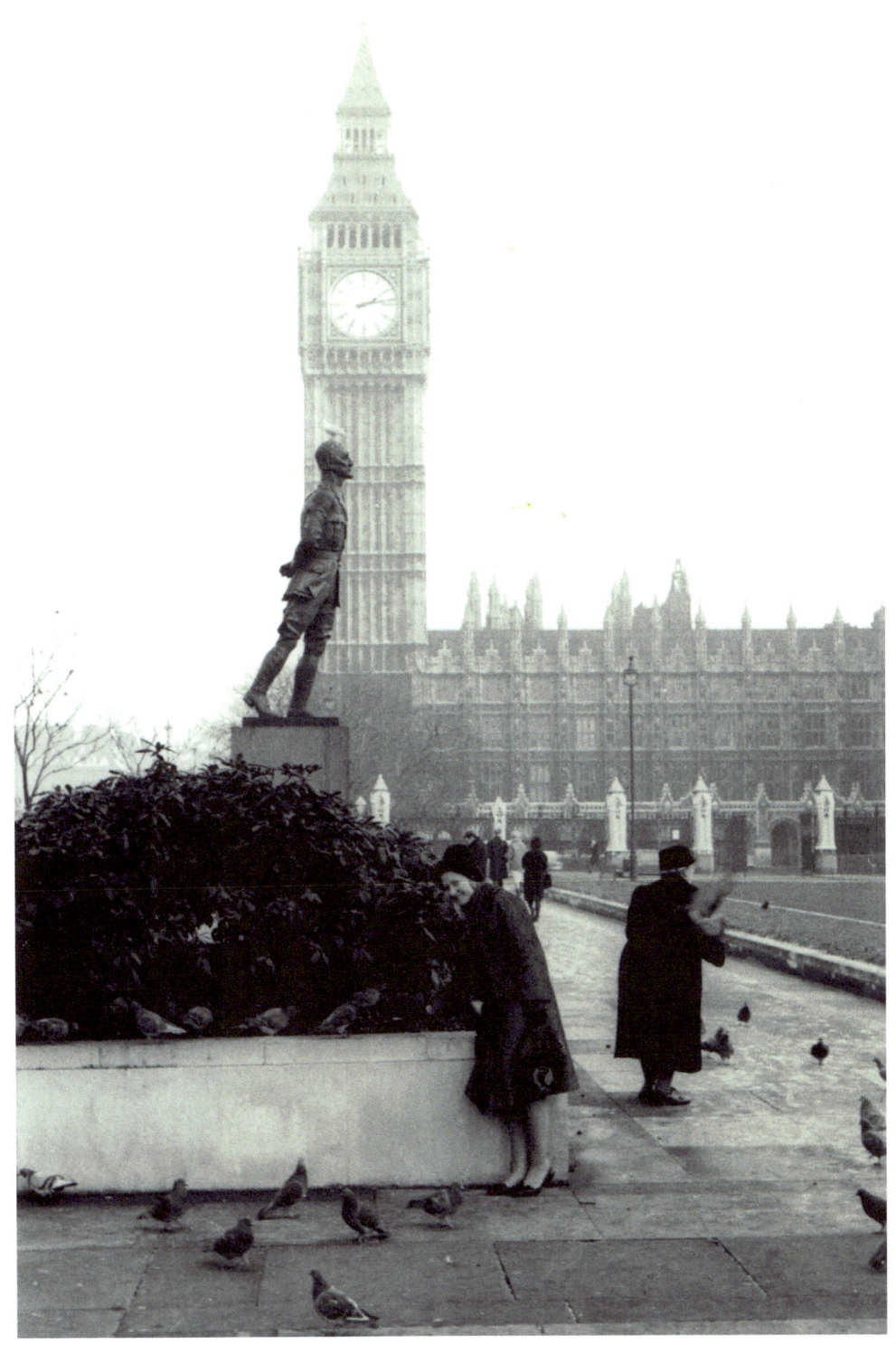

I was a bit at a loss as what to do next. I decided to do a public health course in Amsterdam. This would qualify me to work as a district nurse in my later years as I figured I would not want to work in a hospital when older. I could live at home and work weekends in the hospital in Buitenveldert close to home to earn my keep.

It was actually quite hard as the course was full-time and I worked most weekends. No time for a social life. I qualified after the twelve months and knew that I could always come back to Holland to work as a district nurse. At the time that seemed important to me.

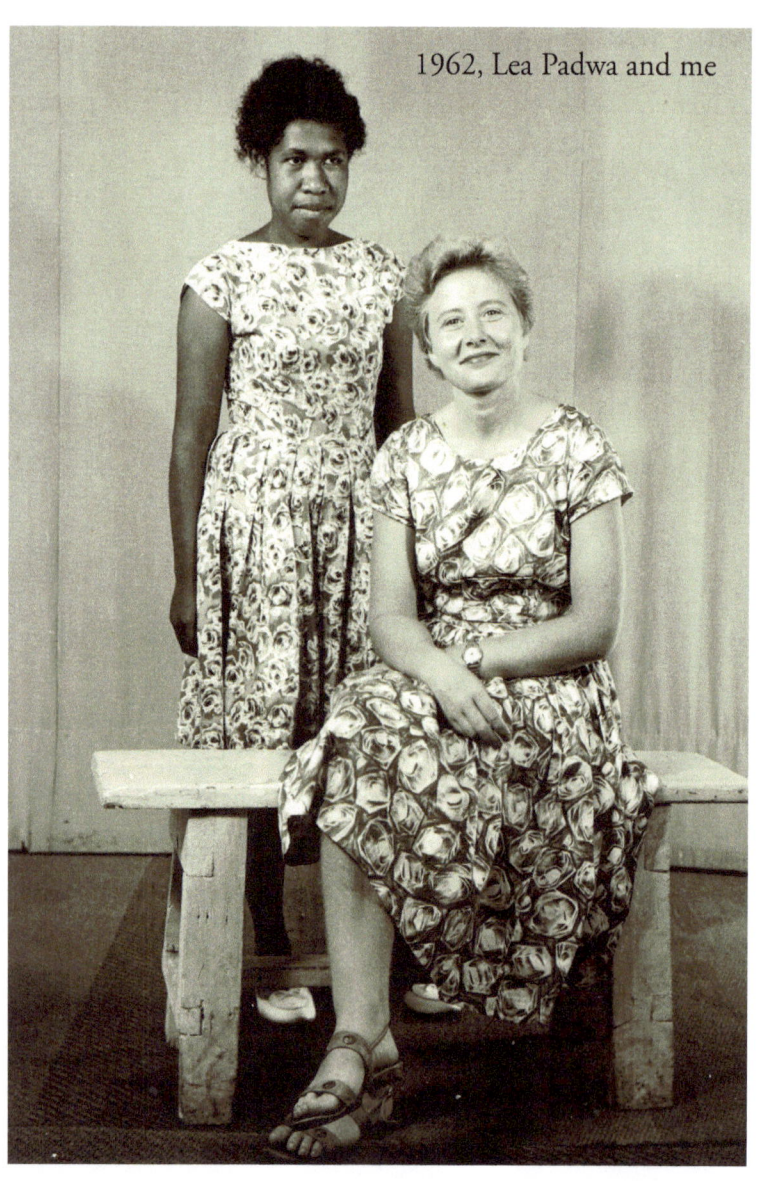

1962, Lea Padwa and me

FRANCE

My friend Els was still in Paris and had married a Frenchman named Jean. We had always kept in touch, and so I decided to go to France. I found a job at the American Hospital of Paris in Neuilly and because I had my theatre certificate I was placed in the theatre. I enjoyed working in the theatre, and I enjoyed Paris on my days off. I often visited Els and Jean and even took horse riding lessons in the Bois de Boulogne. I liked Paris a lot but found my French was not improving as the French girls I worked with, who were working in the American Hospital, wanted to learn English. The doctors all spoke English and Els always wanted to speak Dutch with me. Of course, working in the theatre, you have no contact with the patients as they are anaesthetised most of the time.

So, after a year I joined the Danish Bureau of Nursing, which was a private nursing bureau. I would be working with patients in their own home. They would only speak French, so I learned to express myself. I found French much harder than English. My first patient was in Neuilly (Paris) where I nursed an old lady with dementia.

My second patient was in Normandy on a farm. I nursed a gentleman with advanced throat cancer. He passed away after six weeks, and then I was sent to Cannes to nurse a very wealthy old lady, who employed three nurses, a cook, a housekeeper and a gardener/chauffeur. We nurses would work one day, then be on call for one day, and then have a day off. On our day off the chauffeur would take us wherever we would like to go on the Cote d'Azur and pick us up later in the day. The cook would ask us girls what we wanted to eat and the housekeeper would do our washing and clean our room. The pay was good too. One would think, this job is so good that you want to stay with it. And it was nice for a while. But after a few months I started to think, is this really what I became a nurse for?

I was still getting the "Nursing Mirror" from England and saw an advertisement about nursing in the sun.

This was for twelve months nursing in Zambia, and I thought, yes! I would like to go to Africa.

So, I applied, got the job which was easy having my English certificates, and left for Kitwe Hospital in Zambia.

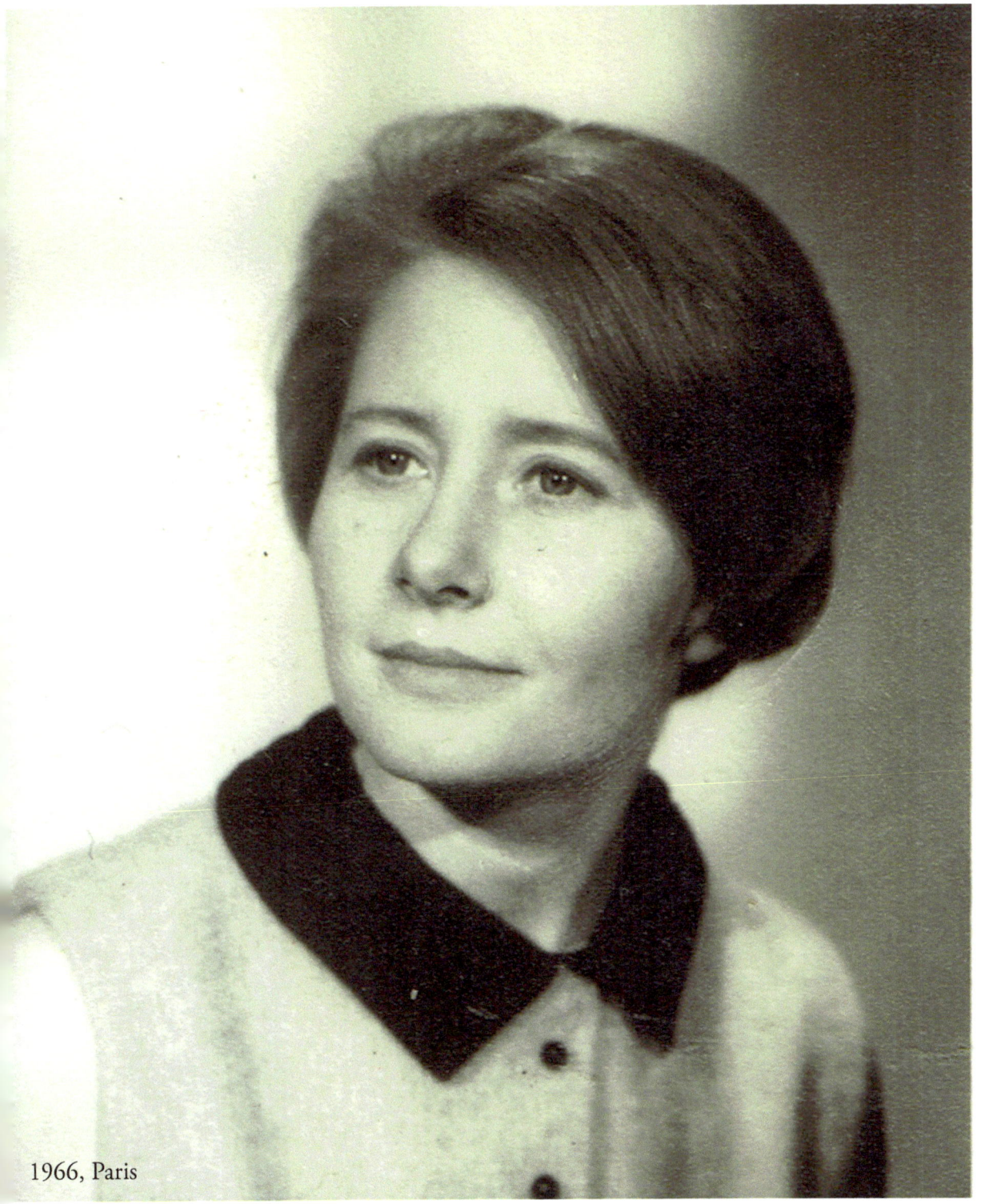
1966, Paris

AFRICA AND BRIAN

I had expected life in Africa to be something similar to life in New Guinea with friendly natives, but I was sorely disappointed.

This was 1966 just after Zambia had become independent under President Kenneth Kaunda. The general population had no idea what independence truly meant. Most thought that they all suddenly would be wealthy and all that the white people owned would now be theirs: houses, farms and cars included. When that did not happen, they became very angry and frustrated.

There was a very strong anti-white feeling amongst the Zambians. People were not friendly. The non-white staff at the hospital were uncooperative. The doctors and qualified nurses were English. The nurses were living in the nurses' quarters at the hospital. I was put on night duty with one African nursing aide on a ward of seventy patients. I was to work from 7 pm until 7 am. The nursing aide, who was supposed to work the same hours, would arrive at 9 pm, put his head down on the table and go to sleep.

I woke him, "come on, you have to help me! There are patients to be changed, drips to be attended to, I need your help."

You know what his answer was? "Do it yourself! You earn twice as much as I do", and he went back to sleep. I was appalled and had to do as much as I could by myself. I could not believe the attitude of some of the personnel. And apparently, they could not be fired.

I was not happy. The food was terrible. I don't know what kind of meat we were given, and no one seemed to know. I think we might have been eating monkey or hyena? It was tough and utterly tasteless.

On my fourth day, Una, a colleague asked me if I wanted to go out as a foursome. Her boyfriend had a friend called Brian, who would be my partner for the evening. I did not know anyone yet, so I agreed. Ted and Brian picked us up from the hospital and took us to a nice restaurant. Una had told me that Brian was a good friend of Ted's and that he was my age. It was a blind date.

I can still see him standing there with an expectant look on his face, which broke into an attractive smile when he saw me.

My first thought? "Hmm, not a bad looking guy".

The dinner went well. I enjoyed the food after the dubious hospital meals. I discovered Brian had two left feet, he was no dancer, but neither was I really unless I had a very good partner. That did not deter Brian from asking me out again the next night and the next.

Then he said he had to go to Ndola for a week. Ndola is another city on the Copper belt. Brian was sales manager for Wilson Rowntree's, the sweets people. As he had a company car to travel for business, he brought his own car around to the hospital for me to use, so I would not have to walk into town in the heat. I was the envy of the nurses. Hardly a week in the country and I had transport! It seemed that Brian had already made up his mind that I was the girl he was going to marry.

Brian loved cricket and all sports and invited me to come and watch him play. I had never seen the game played and did not understand it. I found it boring, and Brian was not good at explaining something from scratch. It was the same with the game bridge. He liked card games, and I did not have a clue. He tried to explain the game to me, but I did not get it.

So I told him that I did not think we had much in common.

He asked, "do you like theatre and music?" So, he took me to see the Mikado, which happened to play in Kitwe at the time. We both enjoyed it very much.

And of course, we both enjoyed travel and camping and fishing. Although Brian had no patience when fishing. If he did not get a bite within the first ten minutes, he would want to move to another spot. As I could sit for hours, just enjoying the peace and quiet. So, the first long weekend I had off, Brian took me to Lake Kariba, where we stayed in a beautiful hotel at the edge of the lake. At sunset, the game would come to the lake for a drink. I had never seen game like that! There were zebras, all kinds of antelope, buffalo, elephants and hyenas. It was truly magic! This was the Africa I had dreamed about!

When at the beginning of December Brian was told by Wilson Rowntree's that he was being transferred back to South Africa, he asked me to marry him and come with him. I told him honestly that I was not sure, as we had only known each other for four months and I had a contract for a year. He suggested that I see the matron and ask what it would cost to buy out of my contract, which I did. When I told him the cost he said, "no problem, I will gladly pay that. Now is there any other reason why you would not marry me? I know you are not happy working at the hospital, so why not come with me?"

I answered, "yes, there is something else, I want you to promise me something.",

"Okay what is it?"

"I want you to promise me that if I ever want a divorce, you won't stand in my way".

He promised and did not at all seem phased by such an odd request.

I had, of course, told him about my previous experience with Will in New Guinea, but that did not put him off either. He was so happy and wanted to ring his mum in Cape Town. We were in the pub at the time, and he yelled into the telephone, "mum! I am getting married! Her name is Cathy, and we will be home a few days after Christmas, so you can all meet her."

We got married on the 24th of December 1966 at a civil ceremony at a friend of Brian's house.

We had about 20 guests, Una and Ted and a few more of Brian's friends and, a few of my colleagues. None of either of our families could attend as it was all so quick and far away.

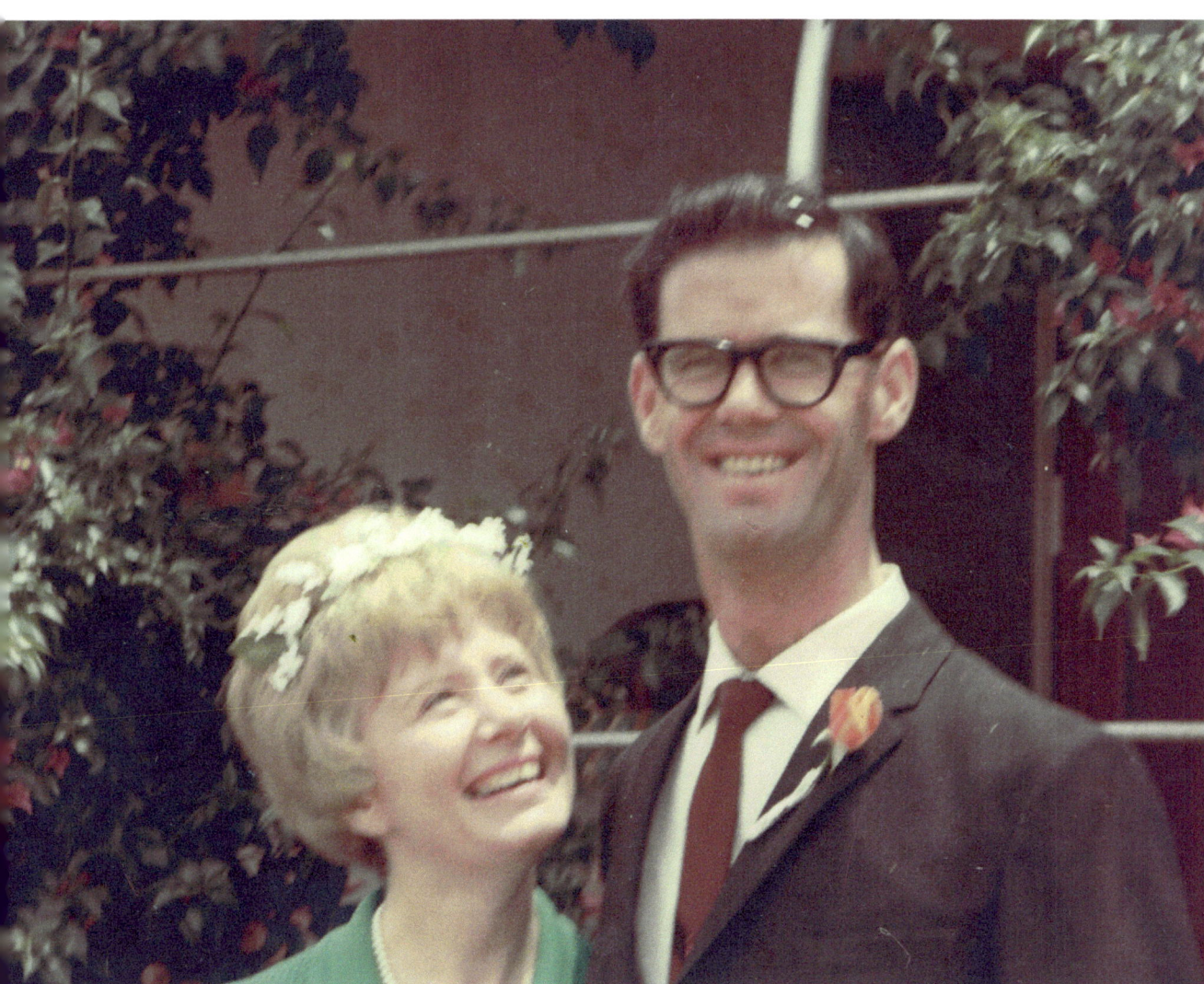

24th December 1966, our wedding day

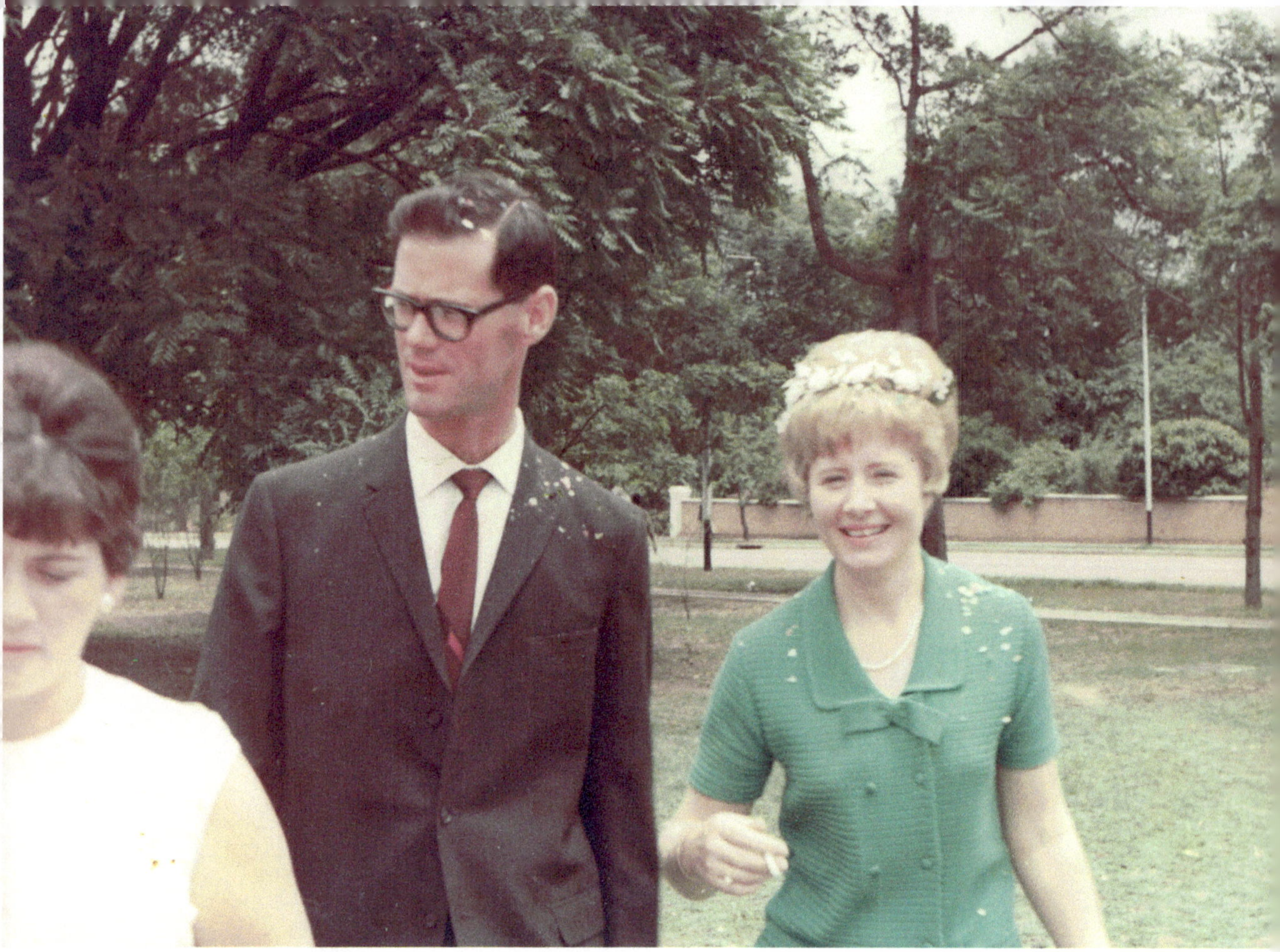

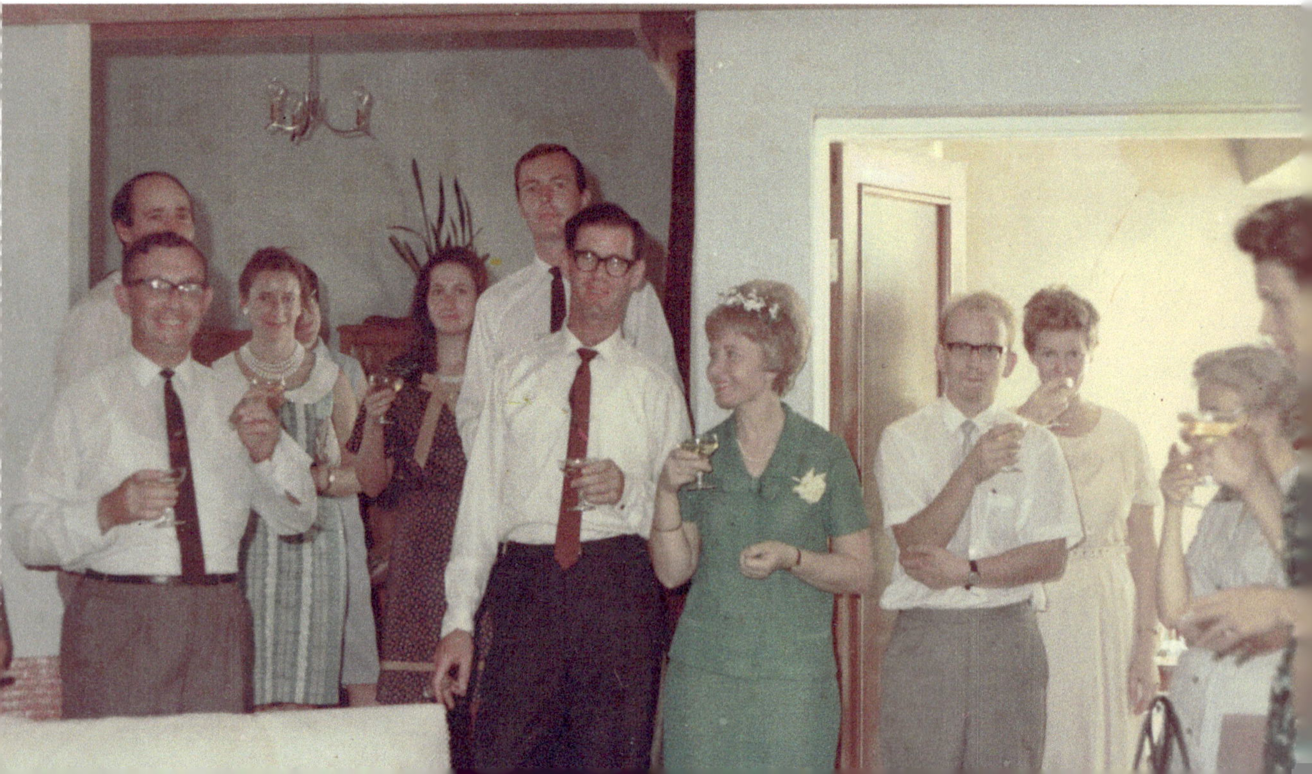

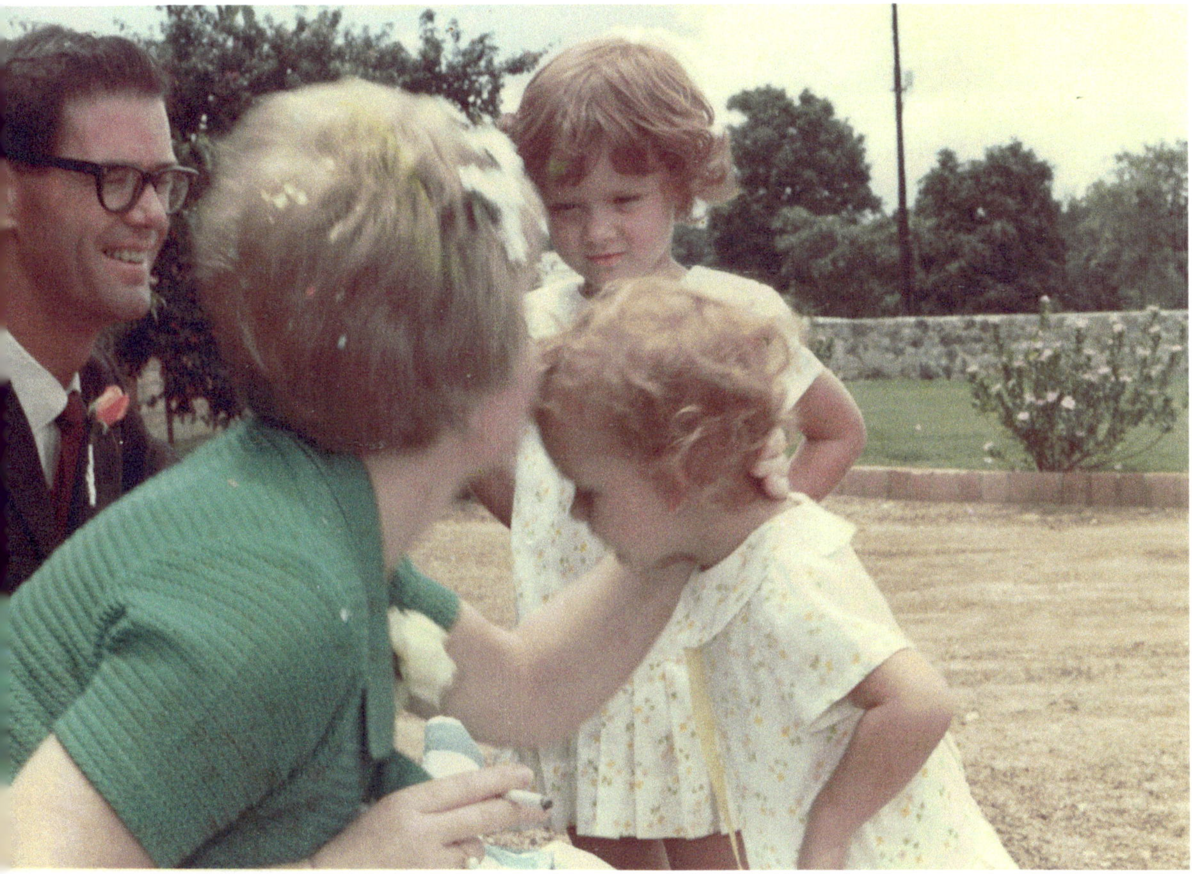

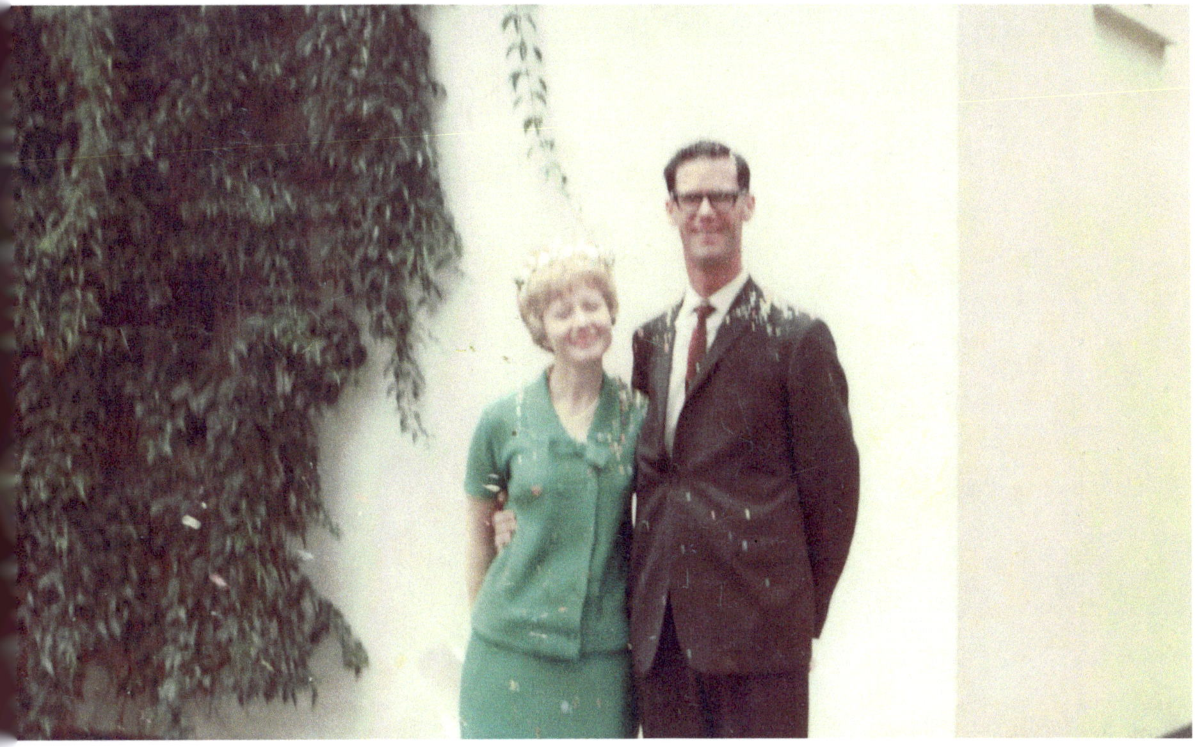

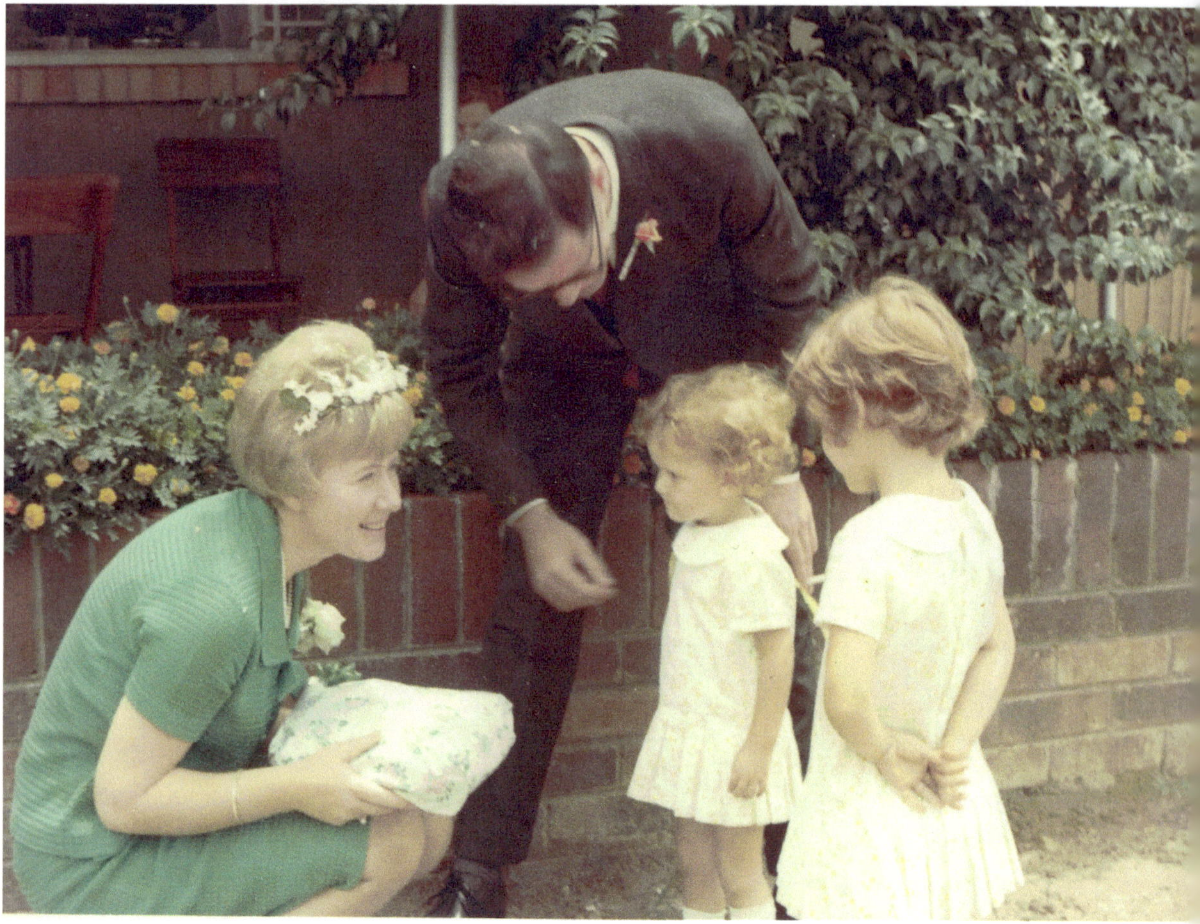

Receiving a gift from Tracy and Gail

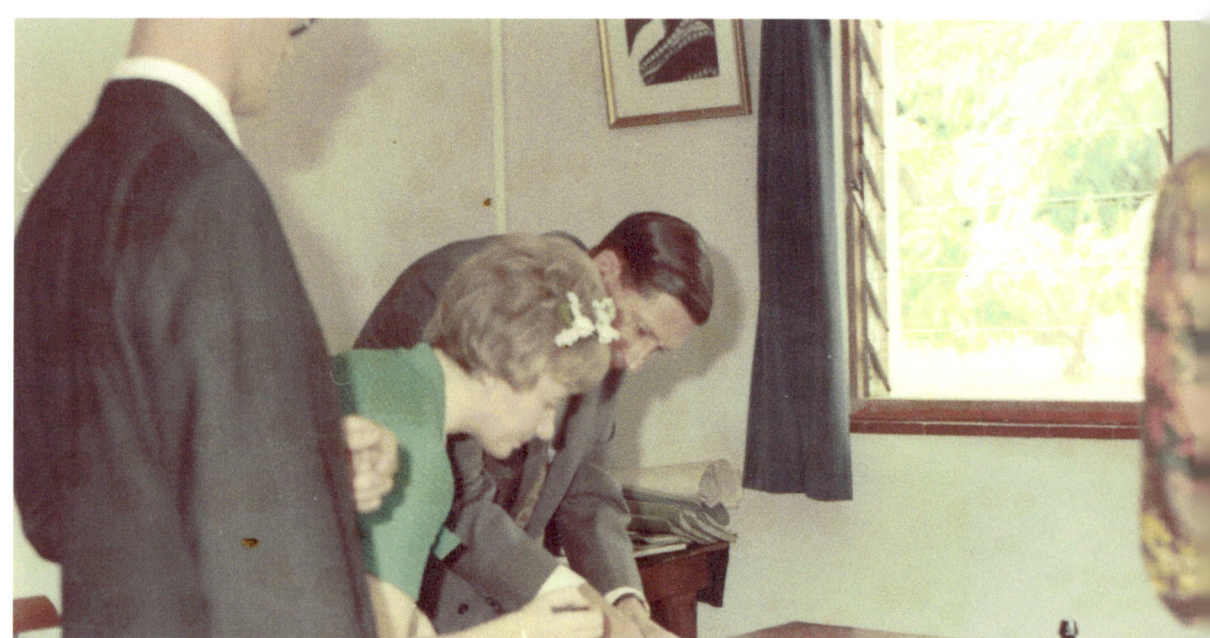

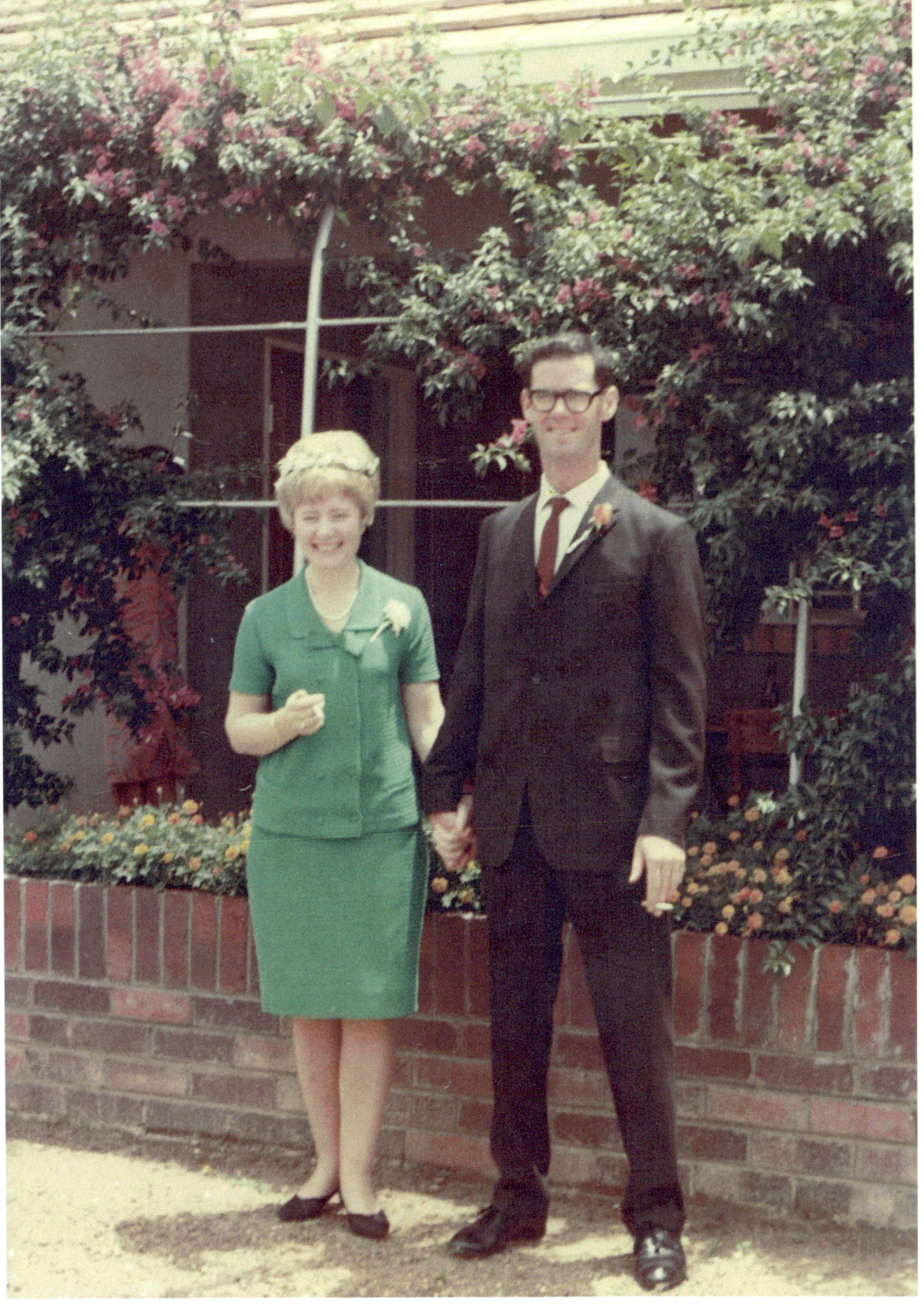

We left Zambia on Boxing Day by car. It was a very long drive to Cape Town, and I was not used to long distance driving. We had left very early in the morning and would drive as far as Leopards Rock in Rhodesia on the first day. After lunch, Brian asked me to take the wheel. I was by then also getting tired, but obliged.

Brian had a nap and when he woke up, told me to speed up as we would not make it to the hotel in time for dinner. I said I would drive as fast as I safely could, which was not fast enough for Brian. Here I got the first taste of Brian's quick temper.

He was suddenly furious and told me to hurry up and go faster. I said, "you drive then because I can't go any faster". The road was full of bends and ravines on one side, and I told him I'd rather get there late than never.

Anyway, by the time we got to the hotel he went to dinner by himself. I was too angry and went to bed. Not an excellent start to a honeymoon!

The next day we drove through Rhodesia and entered South Africa but did not make it to Cape Town. When we got to Cape Town, the whole family was waiting to meet me. Brian's mum welcomed me to the family and everyone was very nice. Then his mum asked me, "Cathy can you sew?" I said, "no I can't sew, when I was at school I tried to learn, but I did not like it."

Then she asked, "can you cook?" I said, "I have not done a lot of cooking" The questions continued, "can you bake?" "No, I can't bake." "Can you crochet or knit?" "No, not really."

By the end of all these questions, I felt totally deflated.

Later when we were alone, Brian noticed that I was upset. "What's wrong Cathy?" he asked me. I told him his mum did not think much of me as I could not do any of the things that are important to his family. He quickly put me right. "Who cares? I don't care; you have so many skills, you are a very highly qualified nurse, you speak several languages, who cares if you can't knit or sew?"

I needed to hear that, but just the same I was glad when we left Cape Town for Kroonstad which would be our home for the next few years.

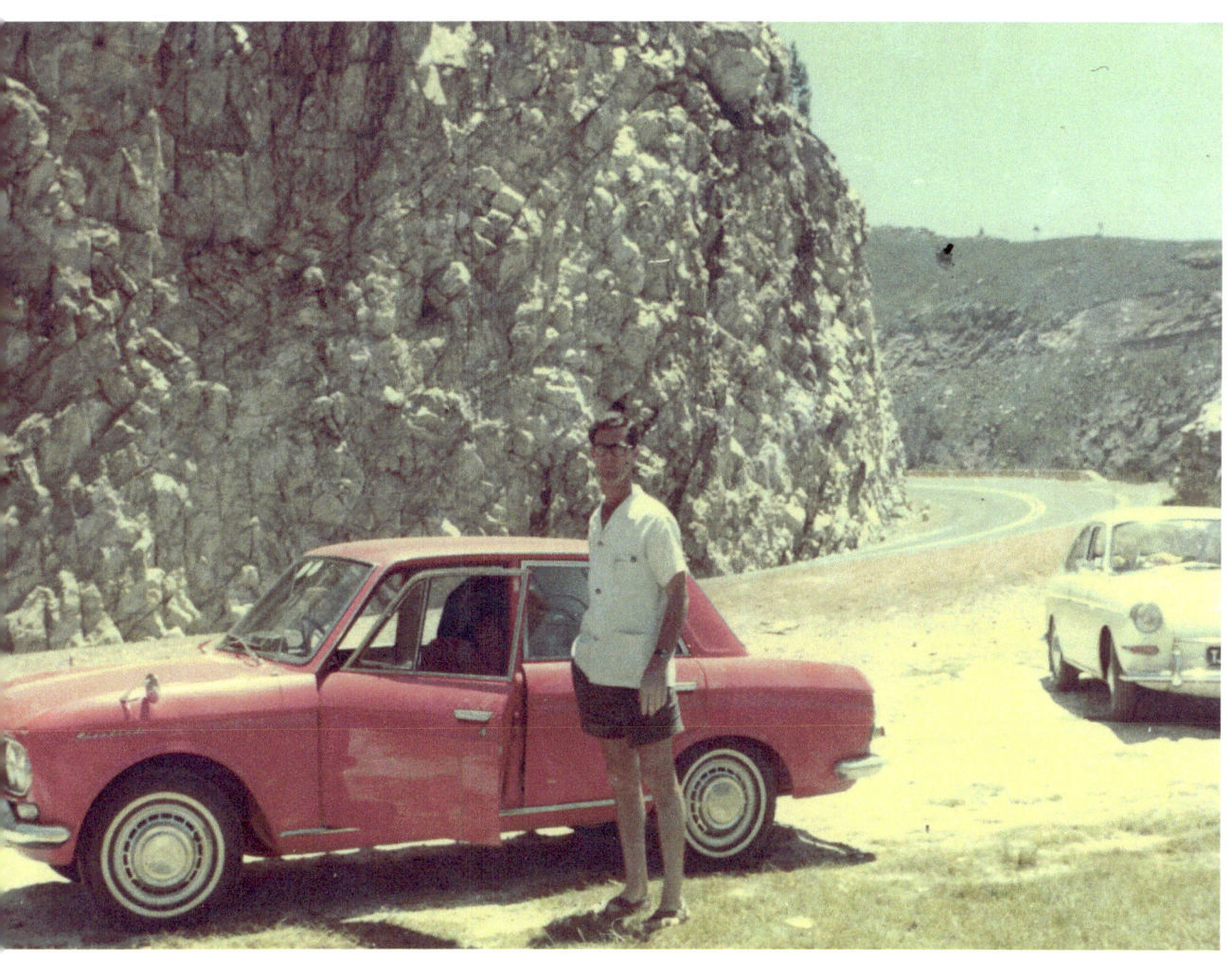
rian and his Datsun

KROONSTAD

We had nothing organised as yet, but as we were looking around Kroonstad, we happened to meet a couple that had a house for rent. They were farmers, named Alec and Lottie Booth. Their mother had moved into town, and the house she used to live in was available if we wanted it. We went to have a look. It was eight miles out of town. We liked it a lot, so now we had a home to move into.

Brian's furniture was already on its way from Kitwe. We only needed to buy a bedroom suite which we could buy in Kroonstad. A whole new adventure began. A brother of Alec's lived close with his wife, Emma. Lionel and Emma became good friends as did Alec and Lottie. They spoke Afrikaans, which did not take me long to learn as it is close to Dutch.

Brian had to travel a lot as he had the whole of the Free State to cover. Having lived on a farm, Brian was keen to start some hobby farming. First, we bought three jersey cows, so we had our own milk supply. We then purchased a separator so that we could make butter and cream. Although I could easily manage the housework, we were told we had to employ a maid for the

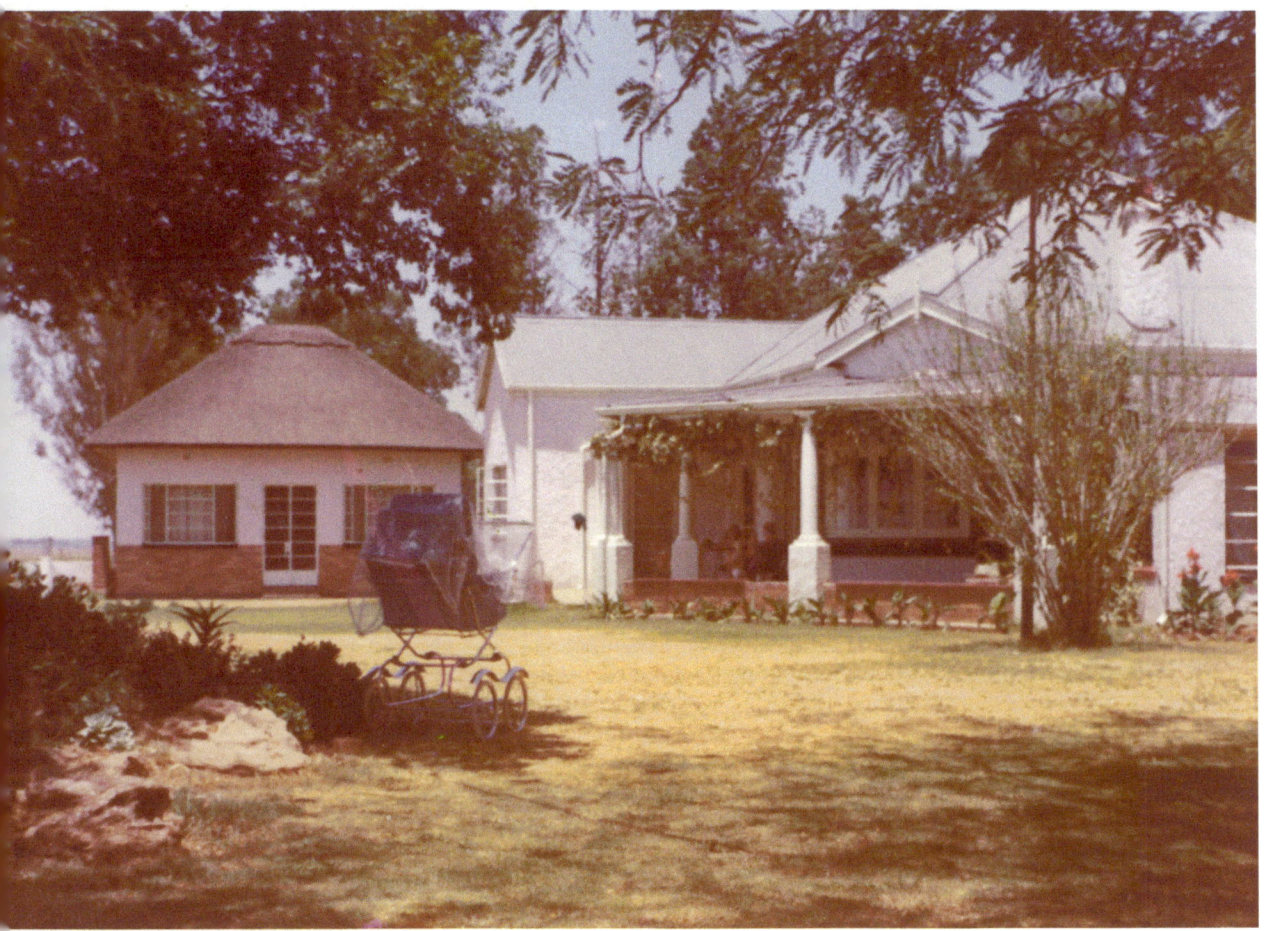

Our house in Kroonstad, Tracy is in the pram

housework and another one for the washing. We also hired some boys to do the milking and keep the yard and garden neat.

As labour was very cheap, it was important for the natives to get a job. One had to provide them with clothes and feed them. At first, it seemed ridiculous to me to employ so many people just for the two of us. As it turned out we needed them.

Alec and Brian decided to start a piggery, so we hired a builder who built the pigsties and then we were ready to buy two sows and a boar and start breeding. It did not take long and the sows were pregnant, and they produced a big litter each. Twelve piglets to one and thirteen to the other. I learned to take out some teeth from each of the piglets, so they didn't hurt the mother when feeding. The boys would do the feeding and cleaning of the sties, but I had to weigh them later on, and once they reached 180 pounds I had to take them to the market and sell them. So now I was a farmer's wife!

What made me very happy was a letter from my mother. She wanted to come and visit us! This was the best news and entirely unexpected. Mum was sixty-eight years old and the only time she had travelled was two years ago when she went to Canada to visit my brother Fons and his wife, Nel. For the first time in her life, she had an income of her own! From age sixty-five she got the age pension. As she lived with my sister Ans and family, they shared the rent and bills, so she was able to save! A friend of Riet named Ali wanted to come with her. Was that O.K.? Of course! We were ecstatic!

Even our neighbours were excited, and the whole time they were with us was such a happy time. Our neighbours went out of their way, and as mum and Ali both loved playing cards, they were a big hit with Brian as well as the neighbours, who also liked playing cards. Mum and Ali loved living on the

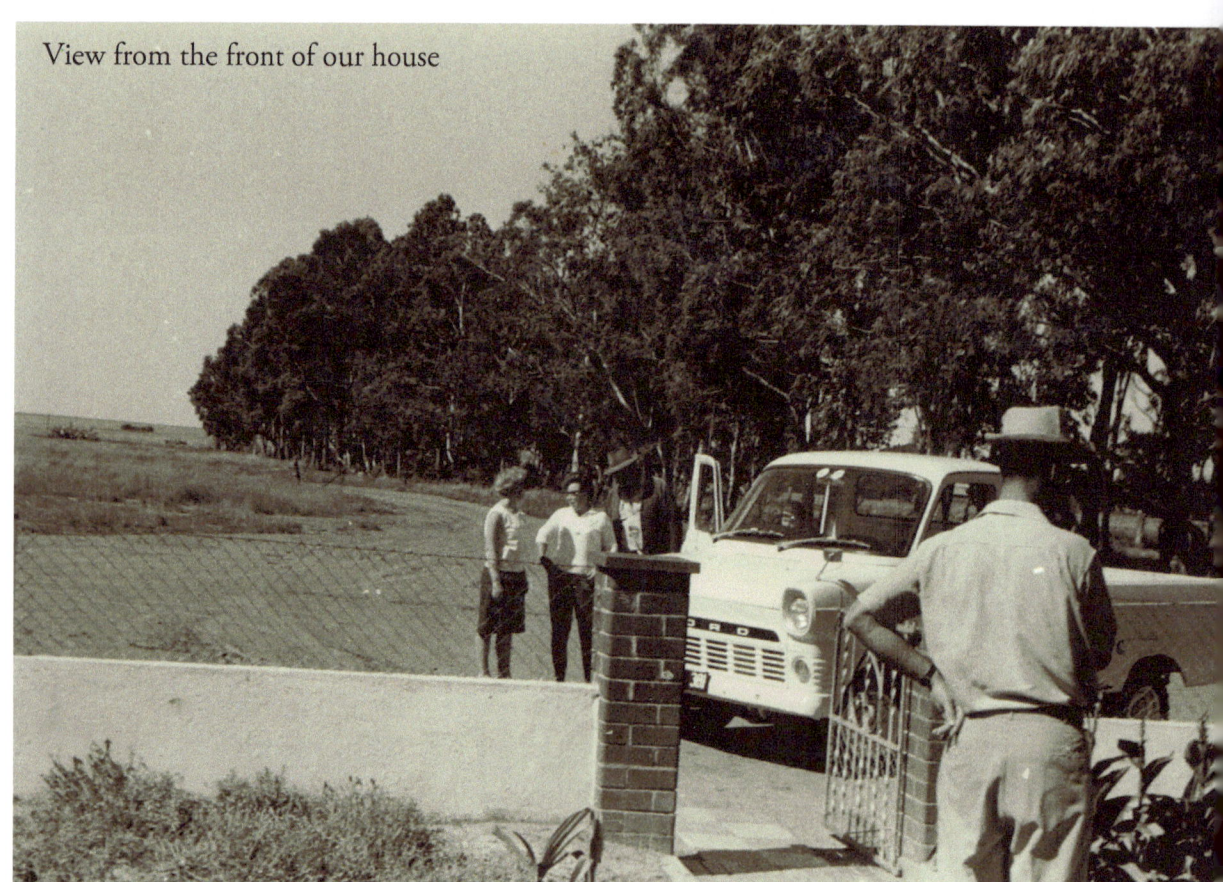

View from the front of our house

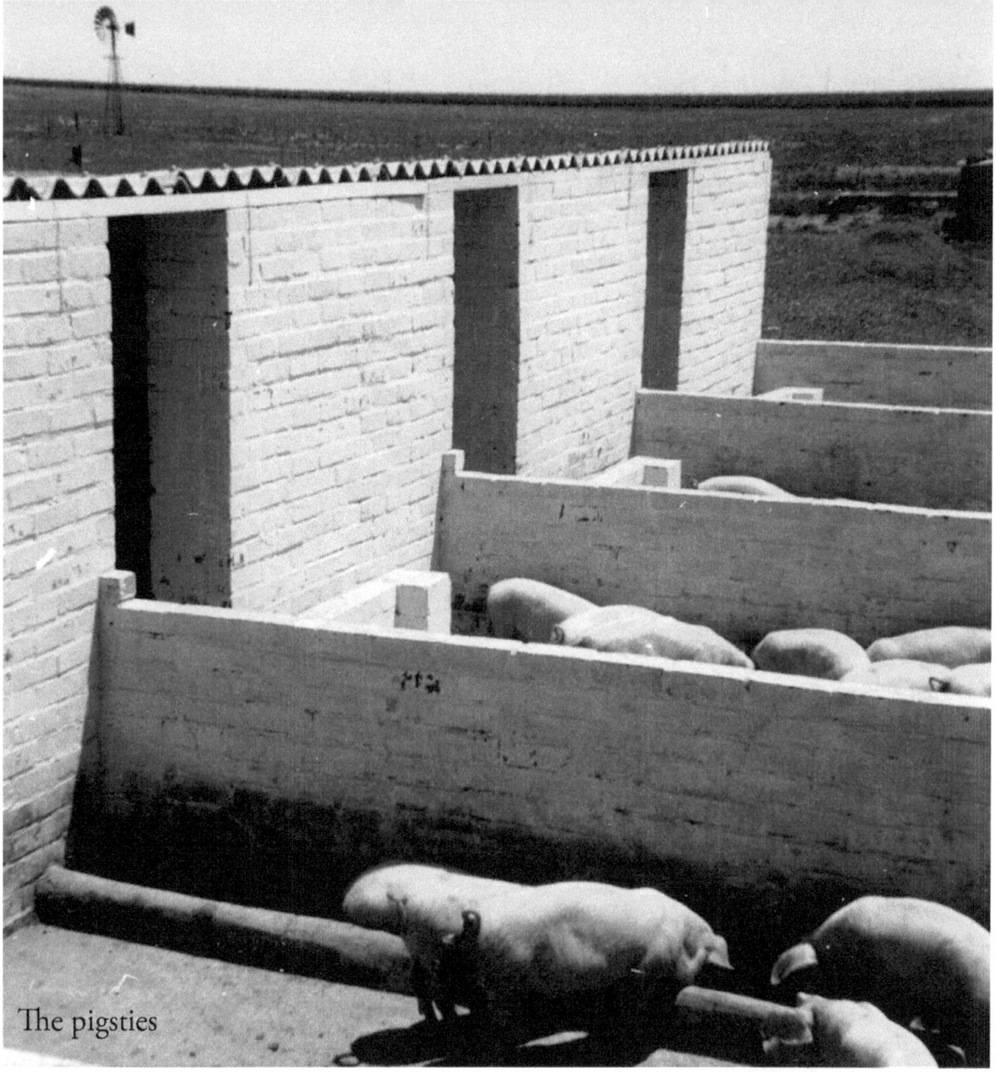

The pigsties

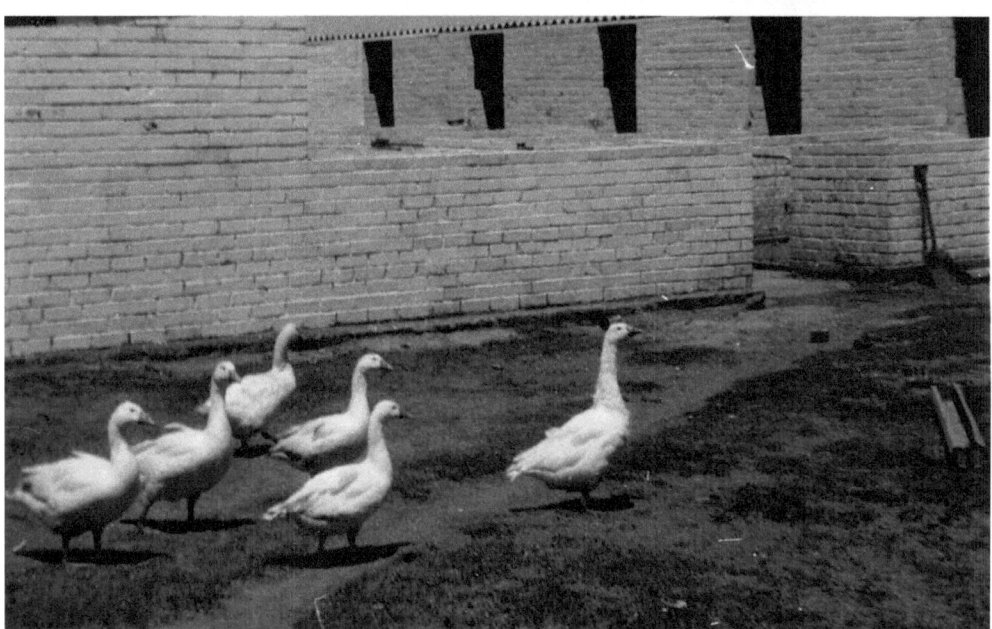

farm and were thrilled when we named the sows after them, Ali and Betsy. The boar was called Elegant. He would allow the children of our friends to sit on his back! Mum and Ali often walked down to the pigs to watch them feed.

They experienced first-hand the famous Afrikaans hospitality bestowed on

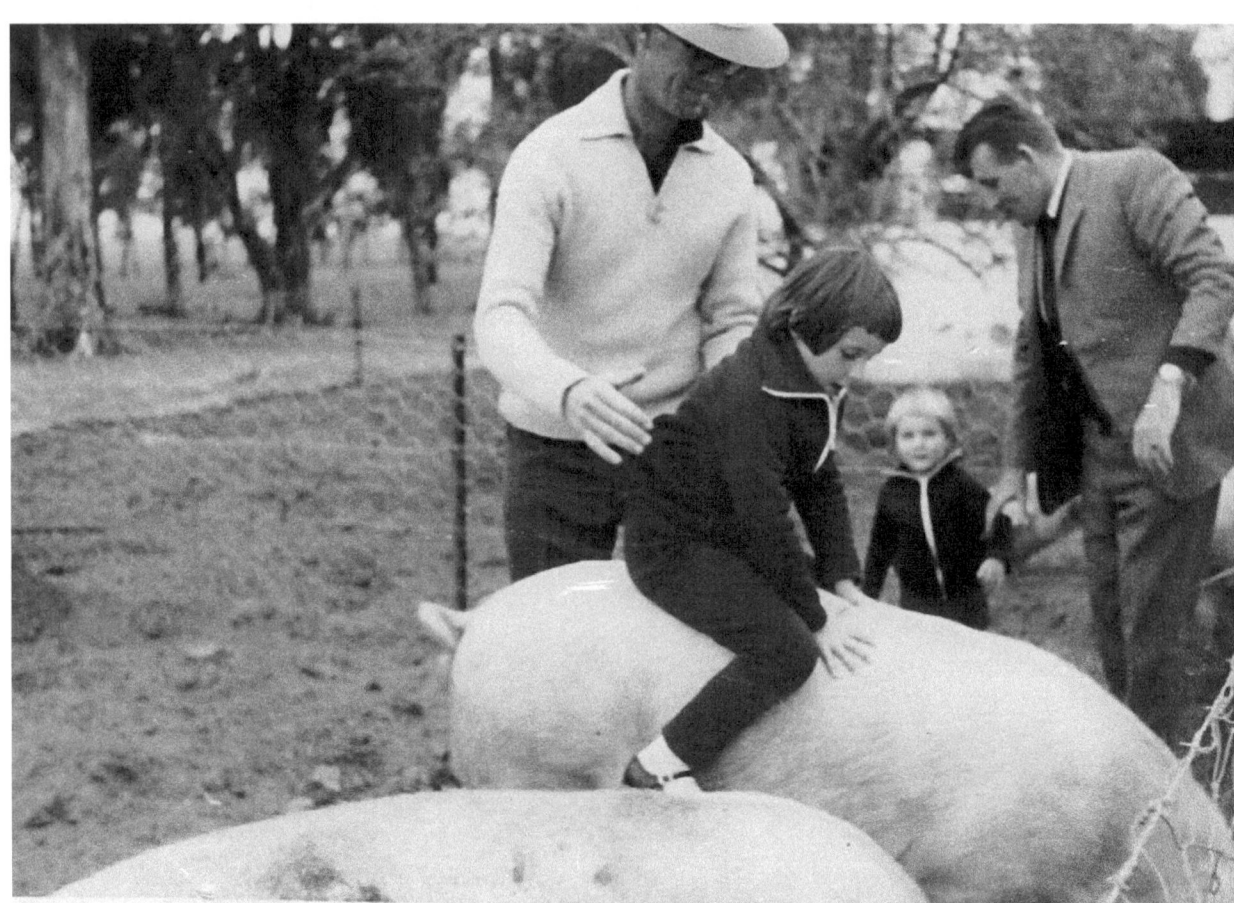

Dianne riding our boar, Elegant

them. Very often we were invited by Lottie and Alec or Emma and Lionel for coffee or tea always accompanied by scones or cake and a game of cards. I kept quite busy learning different skills while living on the farm.

When Emma was bottling fruit or vegetables or making soap, she would call me over to show me. She taught me a lot. The natives that were employed by the farmers in the area, soon found out that I was a nurse. Rather than walking the eight miles into town to see a doctor, they would come to me for advice and help.

My brother in law in Cape Town, who was a GP, sent me lots of samples of medications and ointments and bandages that he got from the various representatives. So I set up an outside room as a treatment room. It took a while to get the people understand that it was not a twenty-four-hour service that I provided, but that they had to come at a specific time unless it was an emergency. I sometimes drove them into town to see a doctor. They did appreciate the free service.

Next thing, Brian decided we should get some chicken and sell the eggs in town. As he never did anything by halves, we ended up with 400 fowls and I would, once a week, drive into town to do the shopping and sell twelve dozen eggs and some dressed chicken. The maids used to do most of the killing and plucking of the chicken as I by now had two children to look after as well as weighing the porkers and taking them to the market.

Tracy had been born on the 31st of August 1968, when I was thirty-five years old. Gerald was born the next year on the 21st of October. Tracy was a very happy, contented baby. She loved to be outside and crawl around the garden, eating my plants. She was particularly fond of pig face (a succulent) and once ate the bulb of one of my amaryllis. She smelled so foul that it took me a while to find out where that smell came from until I found my amaryllis gone. I must not have fed her enough! I had met a friend with a baby the same age as Tracy, who came to play sometimes.

Tracy did not start talking until she was two whereas Gerald spoke in sentences at 18 months.

Being a nurse does not automatically prepare you to be a good mum. In hindsight, I realised that Tracy was so much later to talk because as a small baby I did not speak much to her! I used to feel quite silly talking to her when she could not understand what I was saying yet. Mind you, she has more than made up for those first years.

Brian had bought me a sewing machine, and with much difficulty, I made a few overalls for the children. I hated sewing and still do! I made myself a dressing gown, and that did not turn out too bad, so I decided to make one for

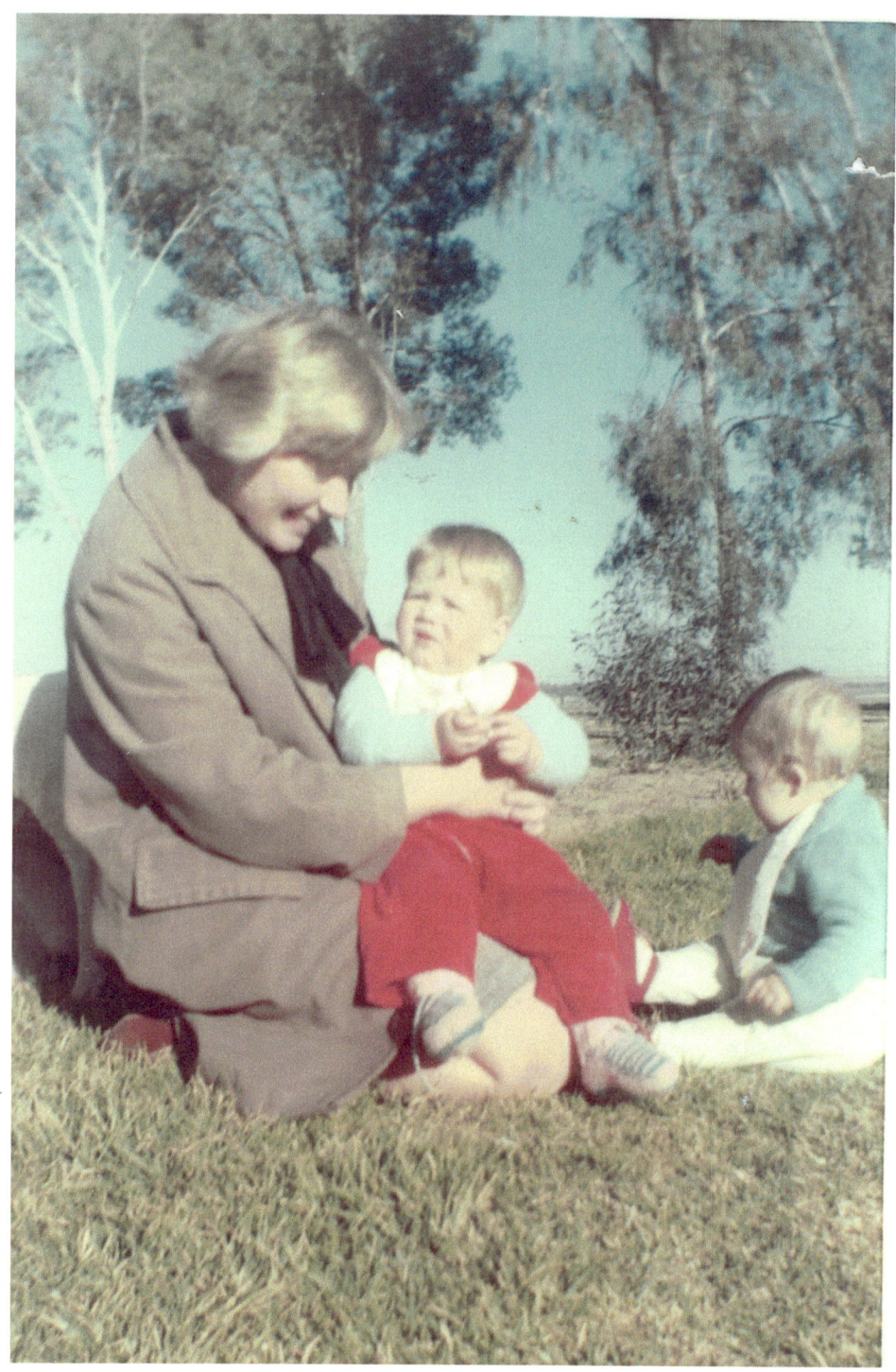

Tracy and me playing in the garden

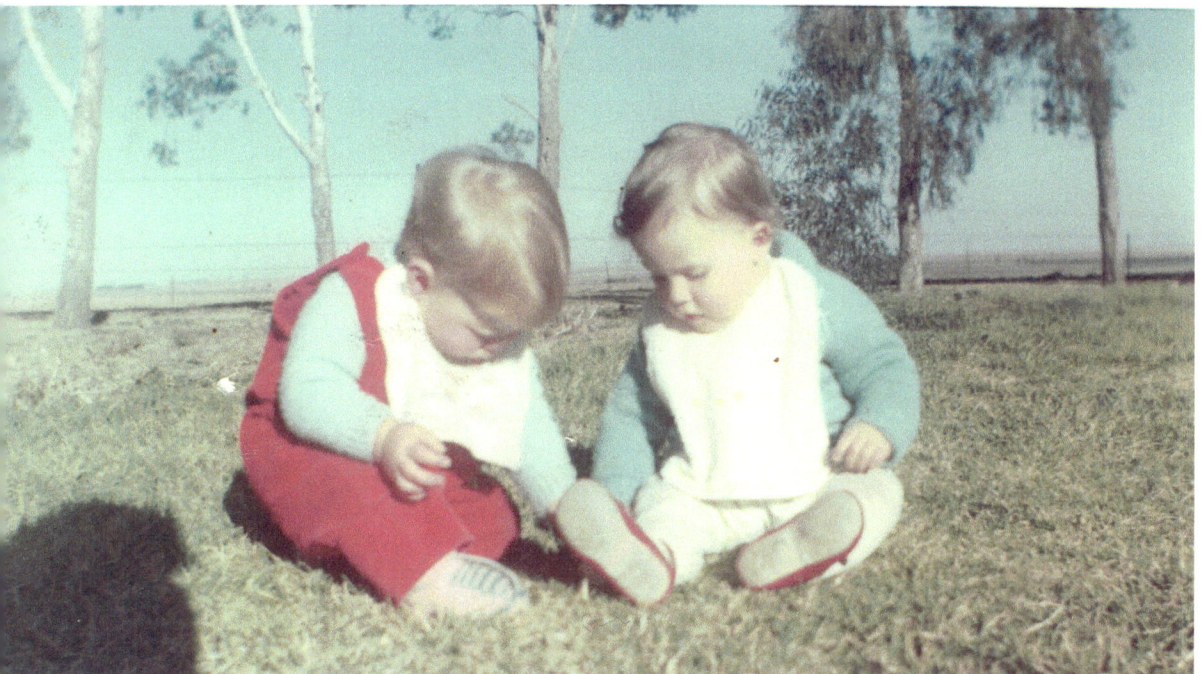

Tracy and her friend

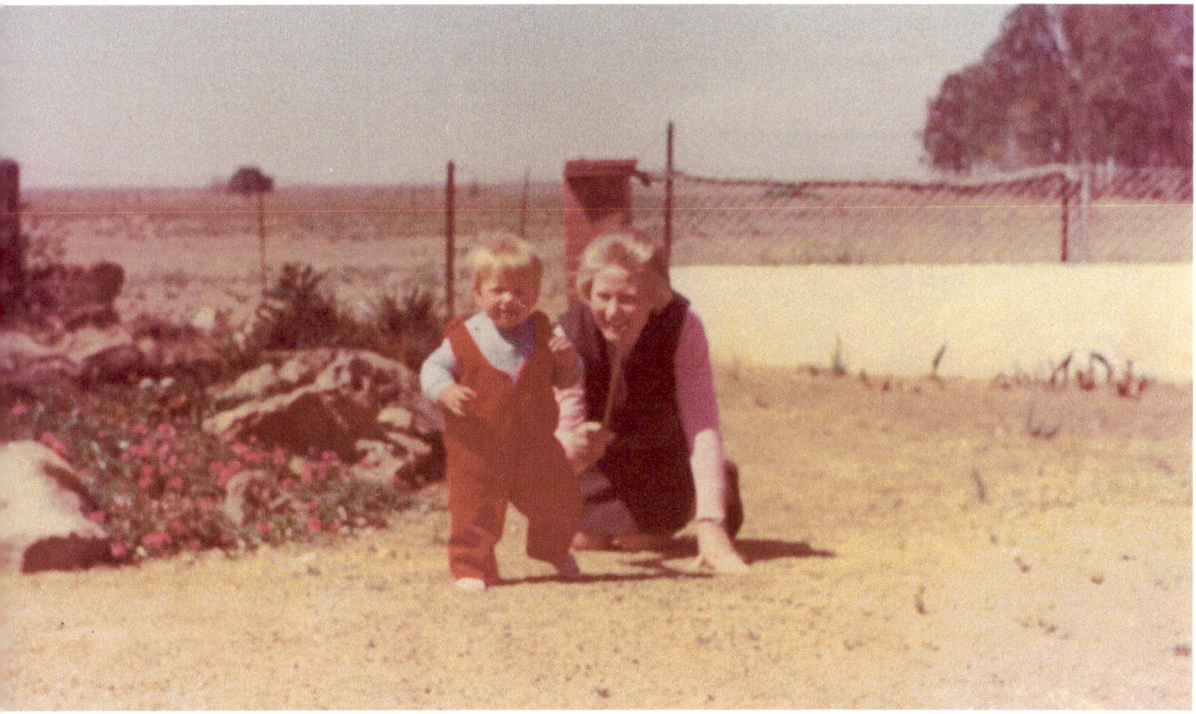

Tracy and me

my mother in law as well. Did I just want to prove a point? I sent it to her as a birthday gift. It must have looked very amateurish. Still a bit sore about my initial meeting? I also taught myself to crochet and made Tracy a little suit, a skirt and jacket. I remember it well.

I must tell you here that I became very close to Brian's mum over the years. She stayed with us many times in South Africa and later visited us several times in Australia. She had such a good sense of humour, and we used to laugh a lot. I loved her dearly!

We often had visitors to stay on the farm. Brian's sister Una had married and lived near Johannesburg. Neil and Una often came to Kroonstad to spend a weekend with us. My sister Riet also came to stay with her husband Jan.

Brian's sister Elin and husband Clive asked if we would have their two children stay with us while they went on a holiday together. Annette, the eldest, was fine, but Helene missed her mum terribly and did cry a lot, especially at bath time at night.

Brian changed jobs and was now working for Denkavit, a company that sold milk powder to dairy farmers. It was more profitable for the farmers to sell the fresh milk and raise the calves on milk powder. The company sent Brian to Holland, Italy and Israel and Brian wanted me to come with him. So the children and I stayed with my family in Holland while Brian went to Italy.

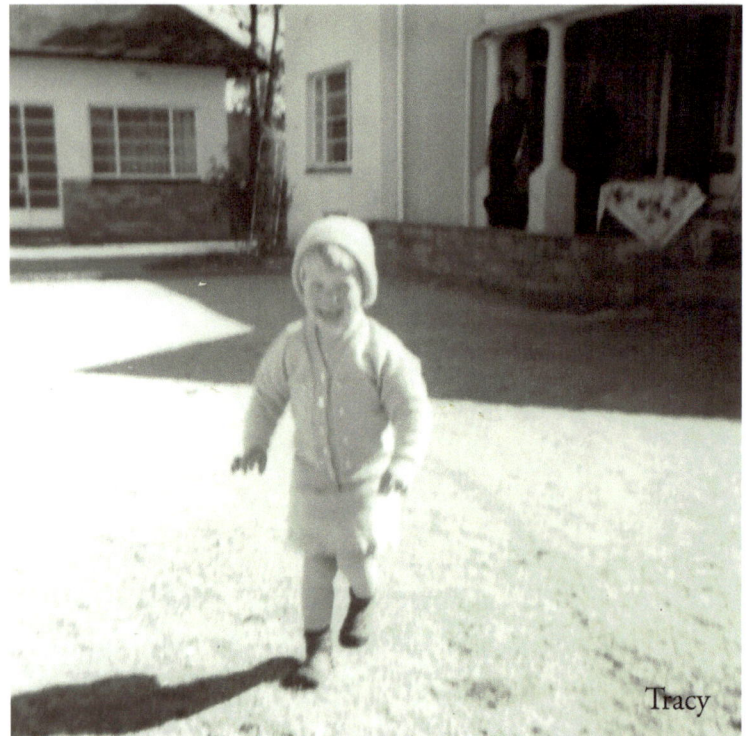
Tracy

Fons, my brother who lived in Canada had managed to come home at the same time with his wife. Good thing the family had moved to a bigger house by now, so we could all fit in.

Gerald had a bad time with an ear infection. Most

likely the result of flying. He was only one year old, and Tracy was two. Gerald cried a lot during those two weeks until his ear infection cleared up.

My big family, Brian (top left) and me (bottom right)

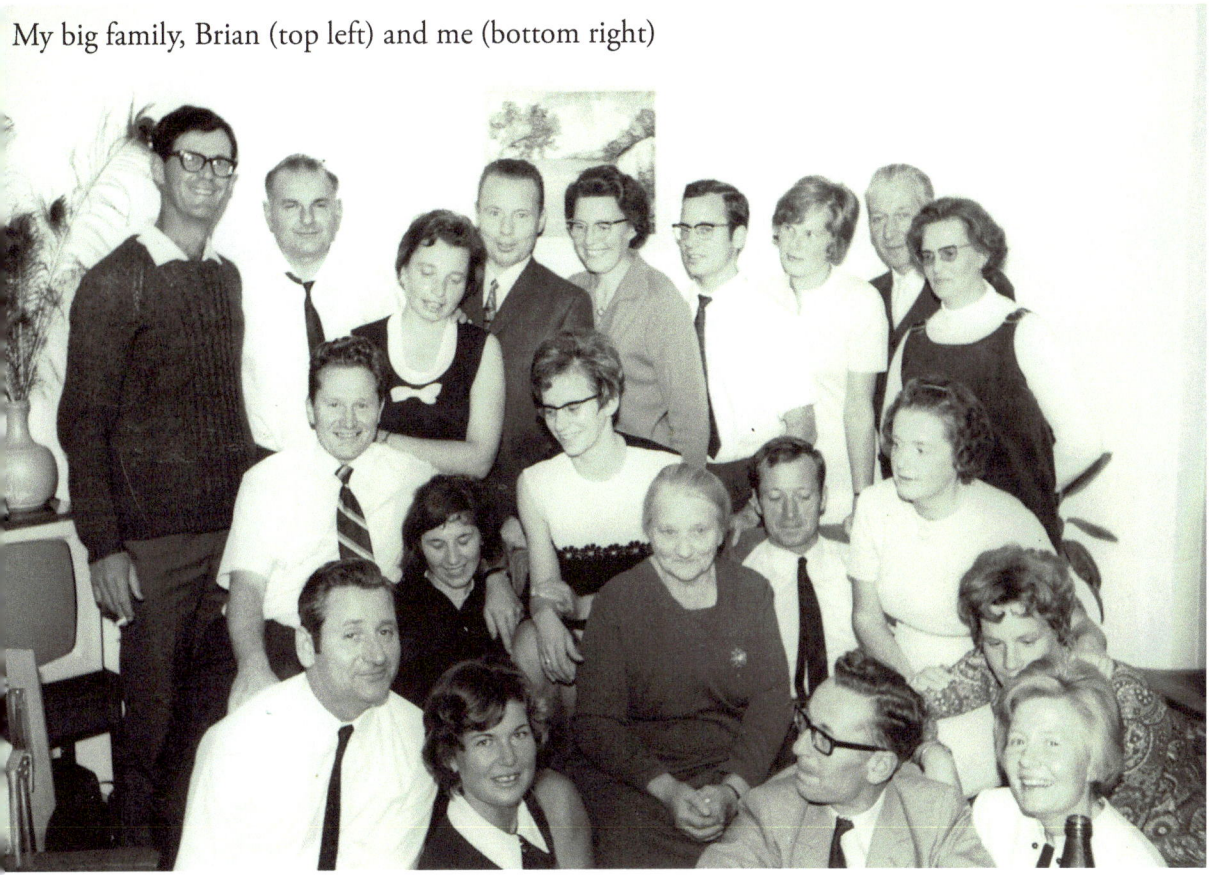

After two weeks we flew to Israel where we stayed in a hotel at the beach in Natanya. We visited a few kibbutzes. We met some very nice people through friends of Brian. The children loved playing at the beach while Brian worked. After Brian finished what he had to do, we had a week's holiday seeing more of Israel, which we all enjoyed. Brian learned a lot about raising calves on milk powder!

Once back in Kroonstad, it was not long before Brian was transferred to Bloemfontein. Although the piggery produced many healthy porkers, which I sold at the Kroonstad market, the price of pork had plummeted. As we were in partnership with Alec, he did not want to continue with the piggery and wanted half of his money, which we did not have. So we owed Alec.

I was pregnant again. We moved to Bloemfontein, where we bought a lovely three bedroom house with Brian's mum's help, as we did not have a deposit. So now we owed Alec and mum.

Mum came over from Cape Town to help look after the children, while I was in the hospital when Wendy was born. Wendy was born on the 12th of June 1971.

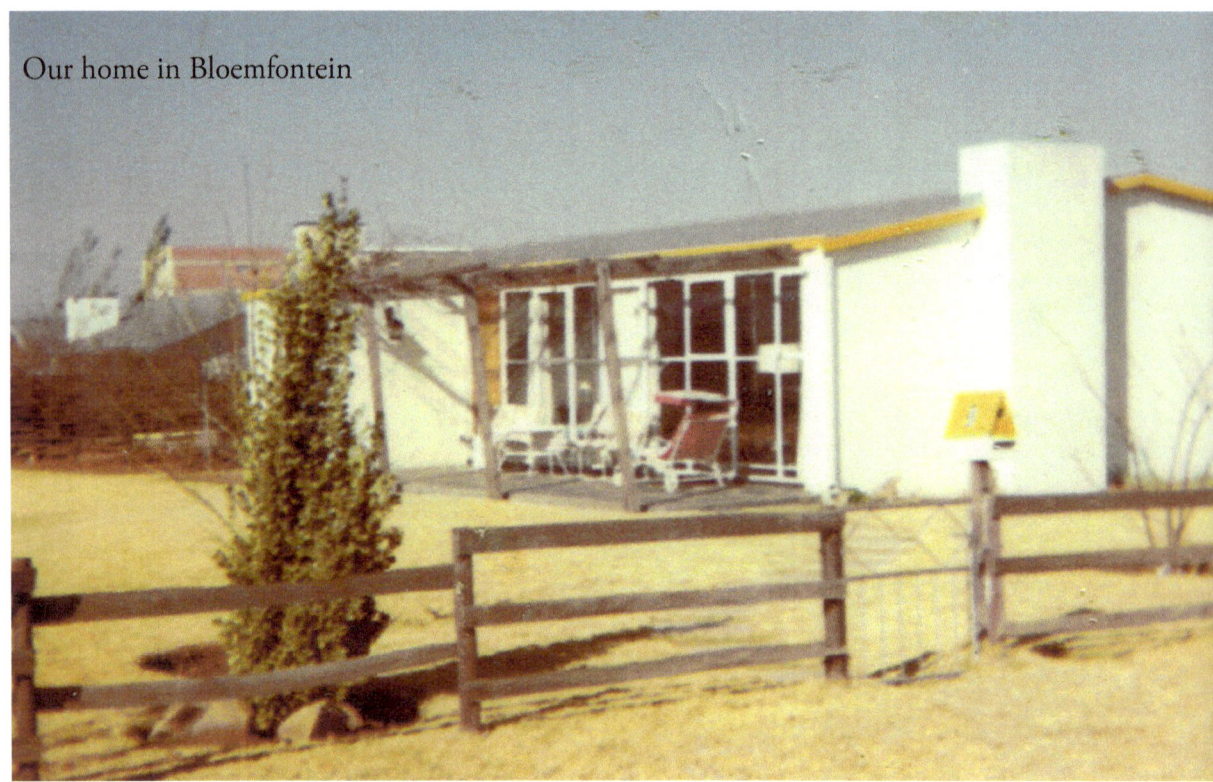

Our home in Bloemfontein

Una and Neil came to visit us in Bloemfontein as did Riet and Jan. When Wendy was four months old, we could see that there was no way we could pay Alec and Mum back unless I went to work.

I had a lot of trouble getting my South African registration, although I had my English certificates. They wanted to know all the details of my Dutch general training. While waiting, I worked as an orderly in the Bloemfontein Hospital in the theatre. I was running patients from and to the theatre. The day my registration came through I was promoted and suddenly worked as a

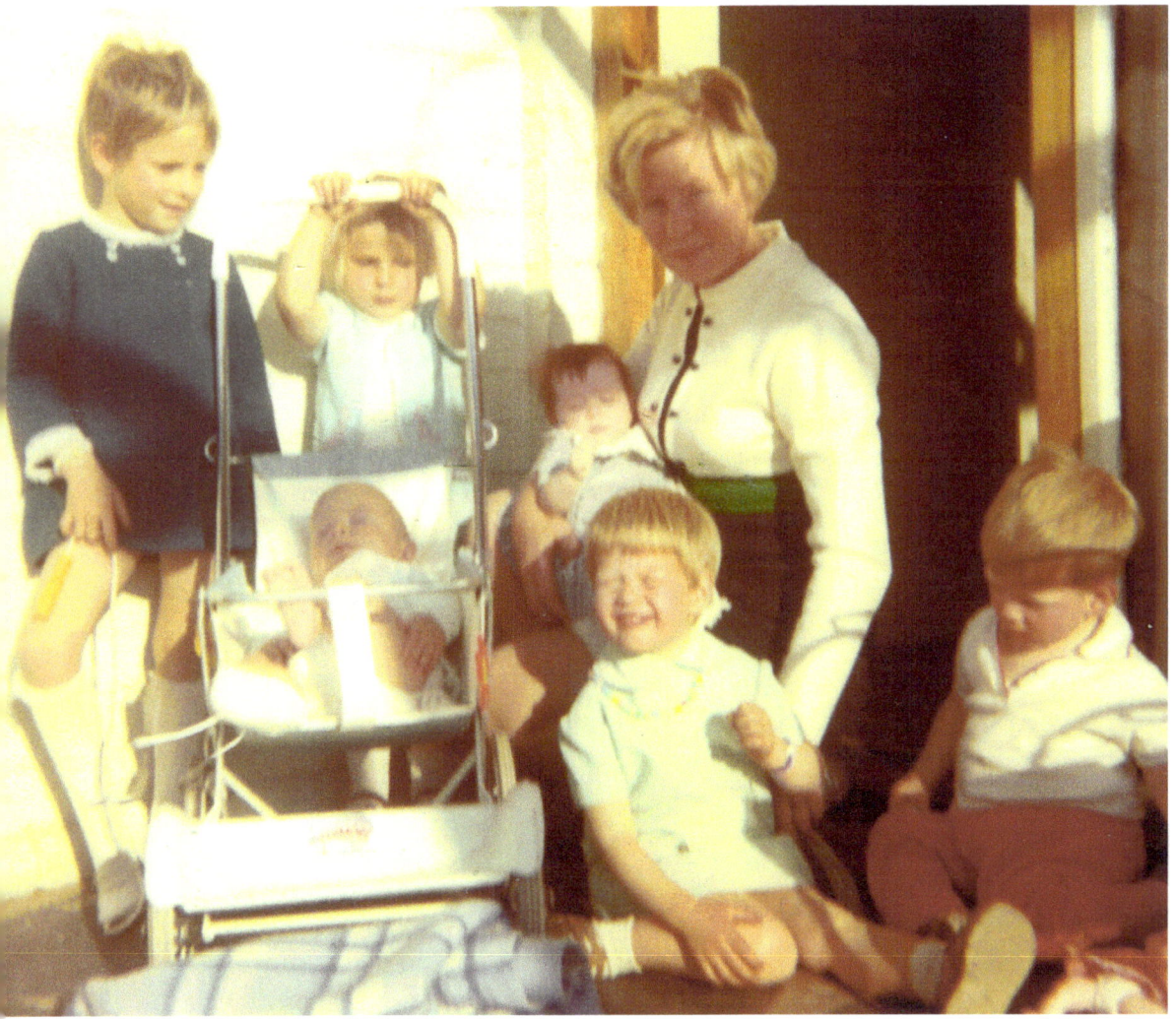

Outside our house in Bloemfontein, Wendy in my arms, Tracy below me and Gerald on the far right, and the neighbour's children

scrub nurse as I had done my theatre training in London.

The hospital had a crèche for the children of staff, but it was a large crèche with sixty children, and our children were very shy. Every morning when I dropped them off, they would cry, and I found it very hard to leave them.

After another four months, Brian was transferred to Paarl, which is a lovely small town about thirty kilometres north of Cape Town in the wine country close to Stellenbosch. We sold our house in Bloemfontein and bought a beautiful four bedroom home in Paarl. This was the only home we have ever lived in that had enough cupboard space. It was built by a builder, who had built it for himself. Every bedroom had large floor to ceiling cupboards, so plenty of room on top for suitcases and camping gear etc.

I very much enjoyed living in Paarl. I got a job at Paarl hospital in the theatre, and the crèche only had twelve children, including our three, with three carers to look after them.

This was so much better than Bloemfontein, and the children were comfortable and happy here. I worked with a girl that also lived in Courtrai (a suburb of Paarl), and she had two children. I used to pick her up and take her home after work. She became a very good friend, and I still keep in touch with Petro and her husband, Faffa Joubert.

I went back to Paarl in 2013 and found the place had changed a lot. I hardly recognised the hospital as it is so much bigger now. It was lovely, however, to catch up with Petro and Faffa, who still live in Paarl. Petro was still doing some relief work. Cecil and Lesley (Brian's youngest brother and his wife) took me to revisit many of the places when I went back in 2013. They still lived in the same house in Durbanville. Since then they have moved to England as life in South Africa is becoming very hard for white people even in Cape Town.

While living in Paarl we often went for drives on the weekend. You could go in a different direction every time within a radius of about fifty kilometres from Cape Town, without repeating the places you visited. There are so many lovely drives! Some along the Atlantic Ocean and some on the Indian Ocean side. The scenery is stunning wherever you venture.

Although we were happy living in Paarl, Brian felt that South Africa was not the country for our children to grow up in. The children were now two and a half, four and five and if we moved we should do it now. Before they had made friends at school and would find it much harder. So we started looking at our options.

We both thought Australia might be a good place. Similar climate, English speaking, stable economy. But would we readily be accepted as migrants?

Luck was on our side as Australia was short of nurses. We were accepted and had to make our own way, so we decided to go by ship.

We sold our house in Paarl, which did not take long. We spent the last month in Elin and Clive's home in Gordon's Bay.

We left Cape Town on the 10th of December 1973 for Fremantle on the Marconi, an Italian migrant ship. The journey took ten days and was not very pleasant as the ocean was rough and a lot of people were seasick.

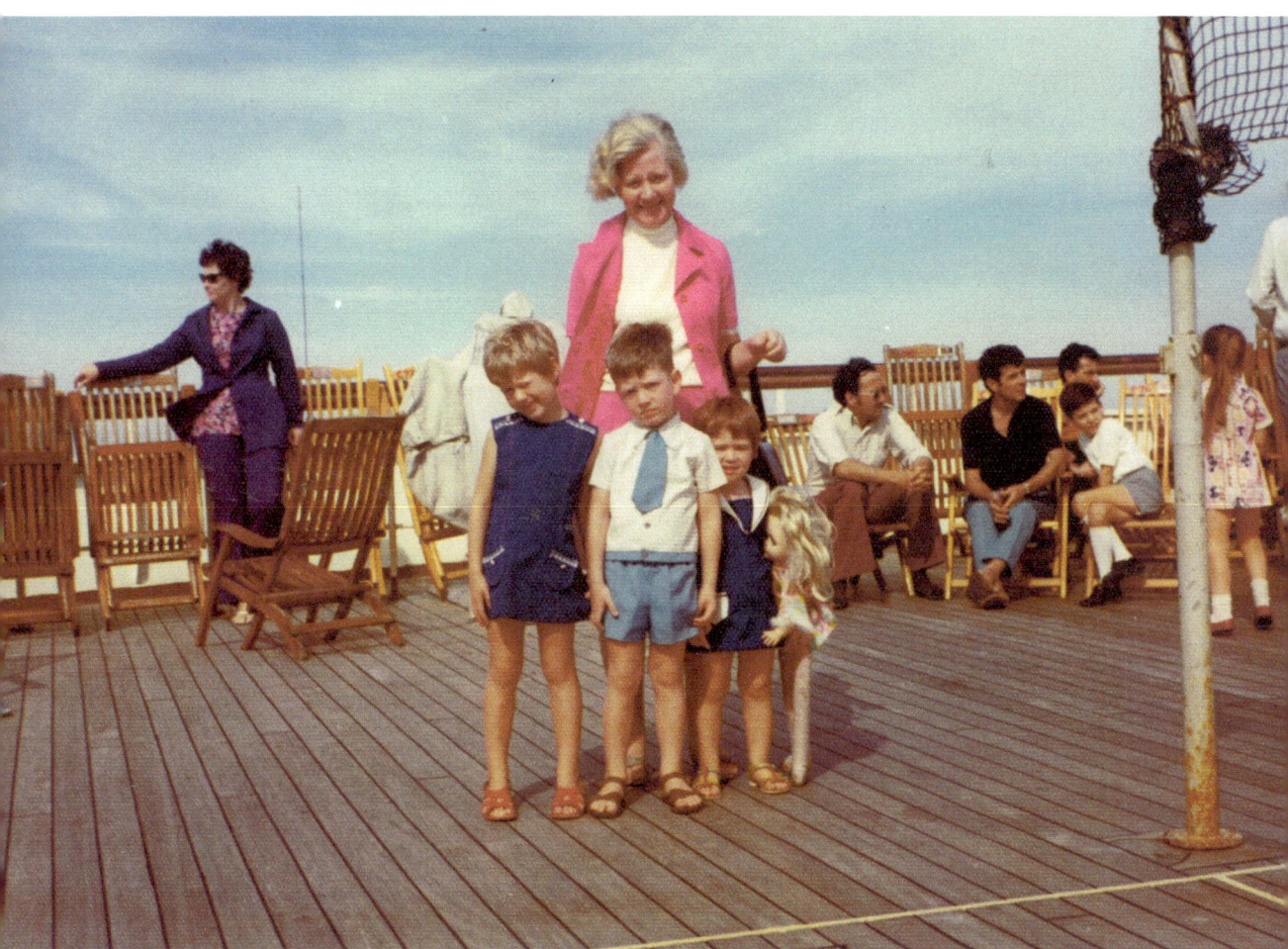

On board the Marconi

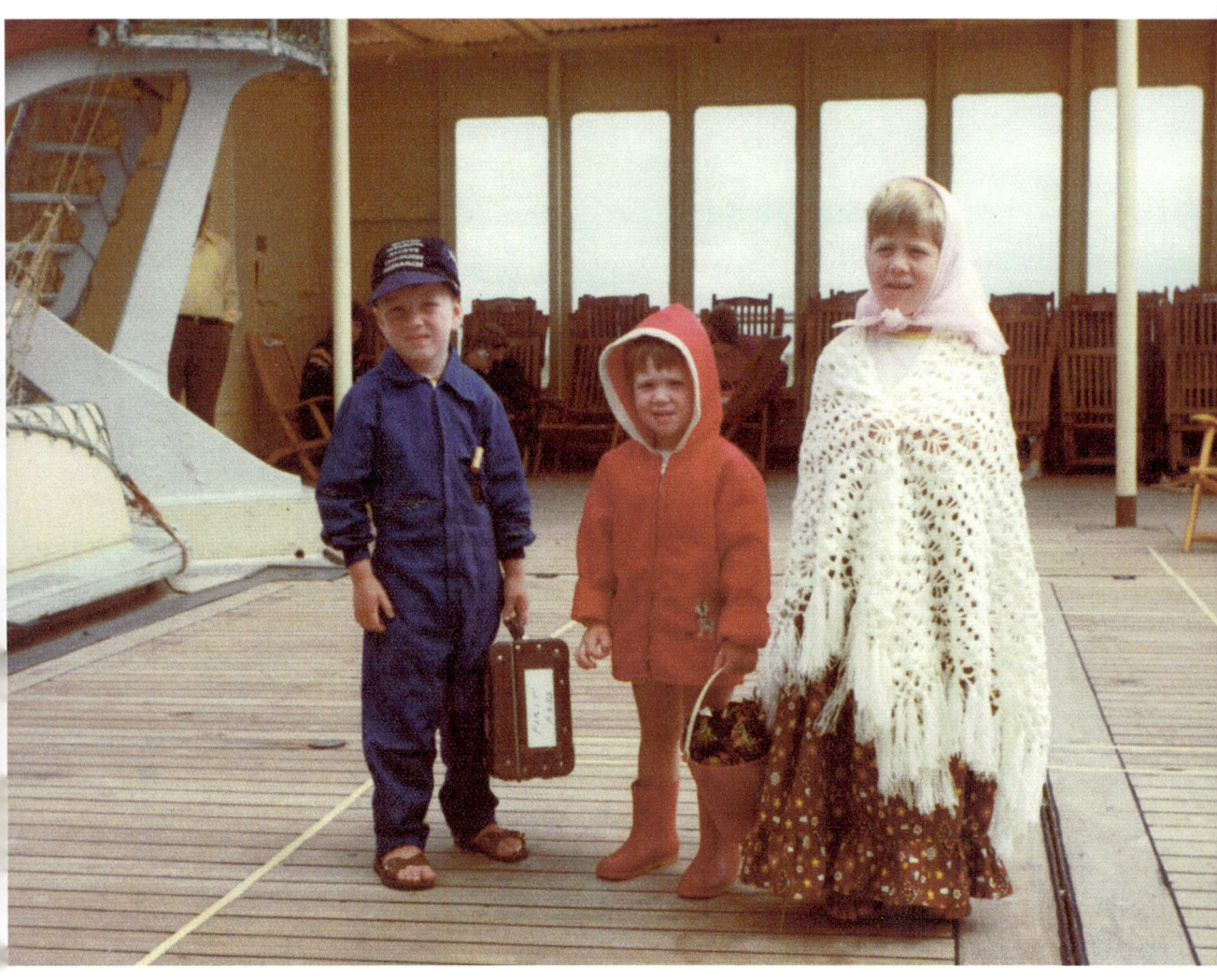

December 1973, a dress up party on board the Marconi to Australia

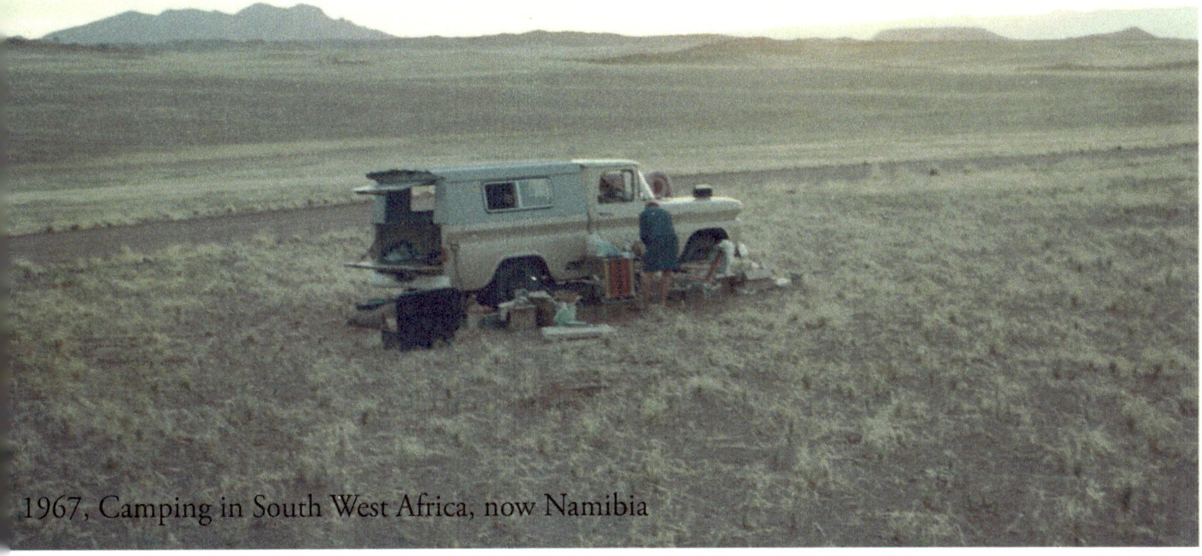

1967, Camping in South West Africa, now Namibia

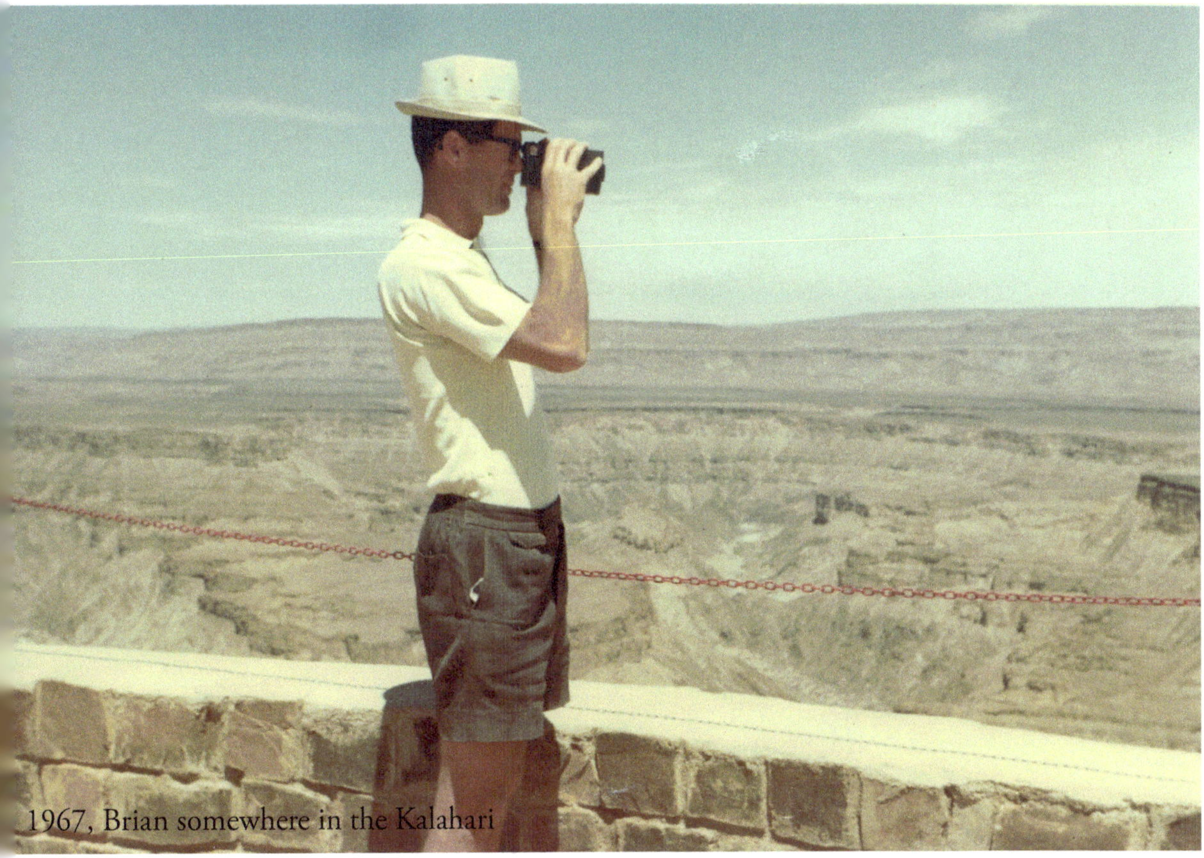

1967, Brian somewhere in the Kalahari

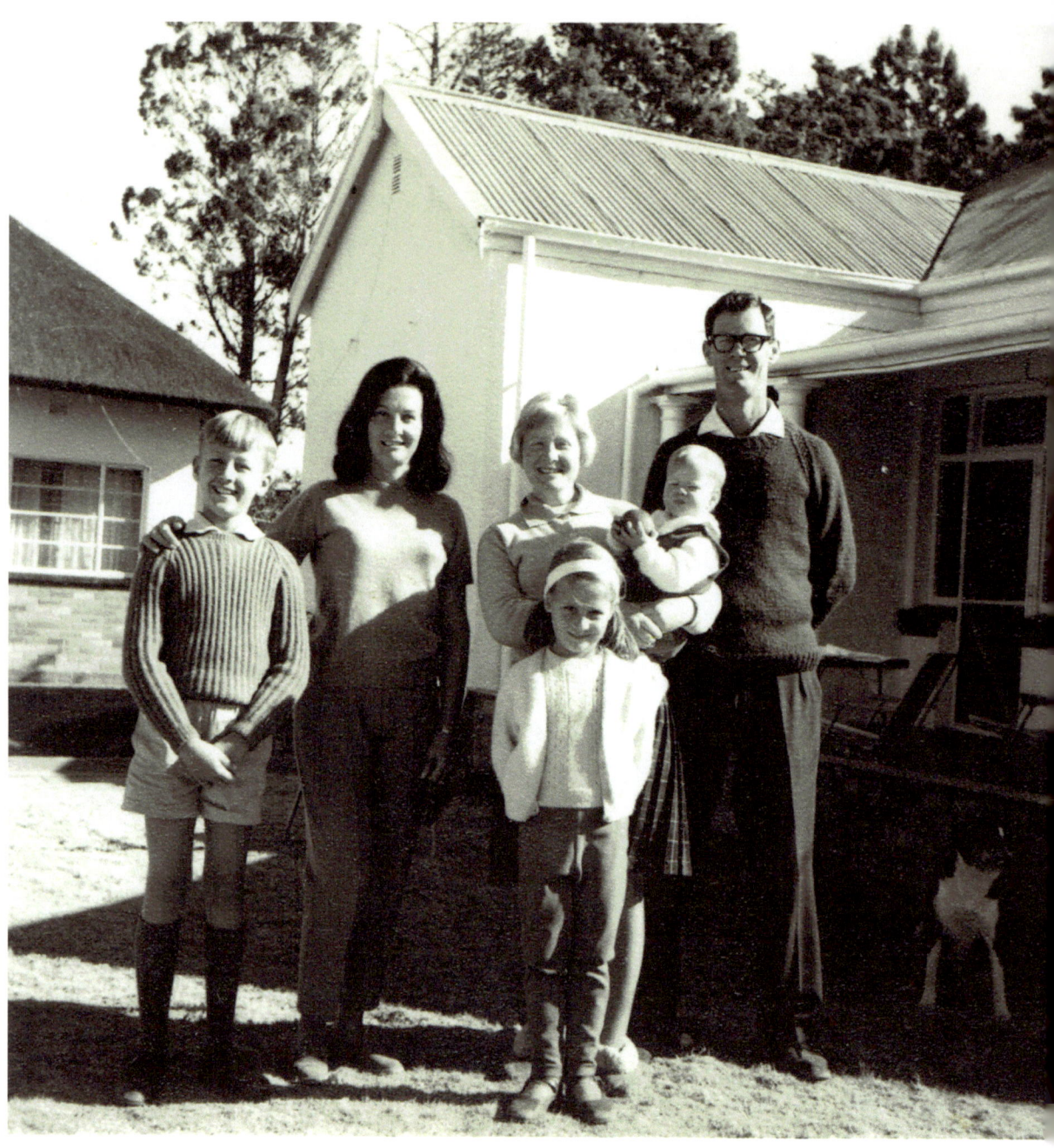

A visit from Earl and Gwenyth Wyssel with their children Russel and Andrea

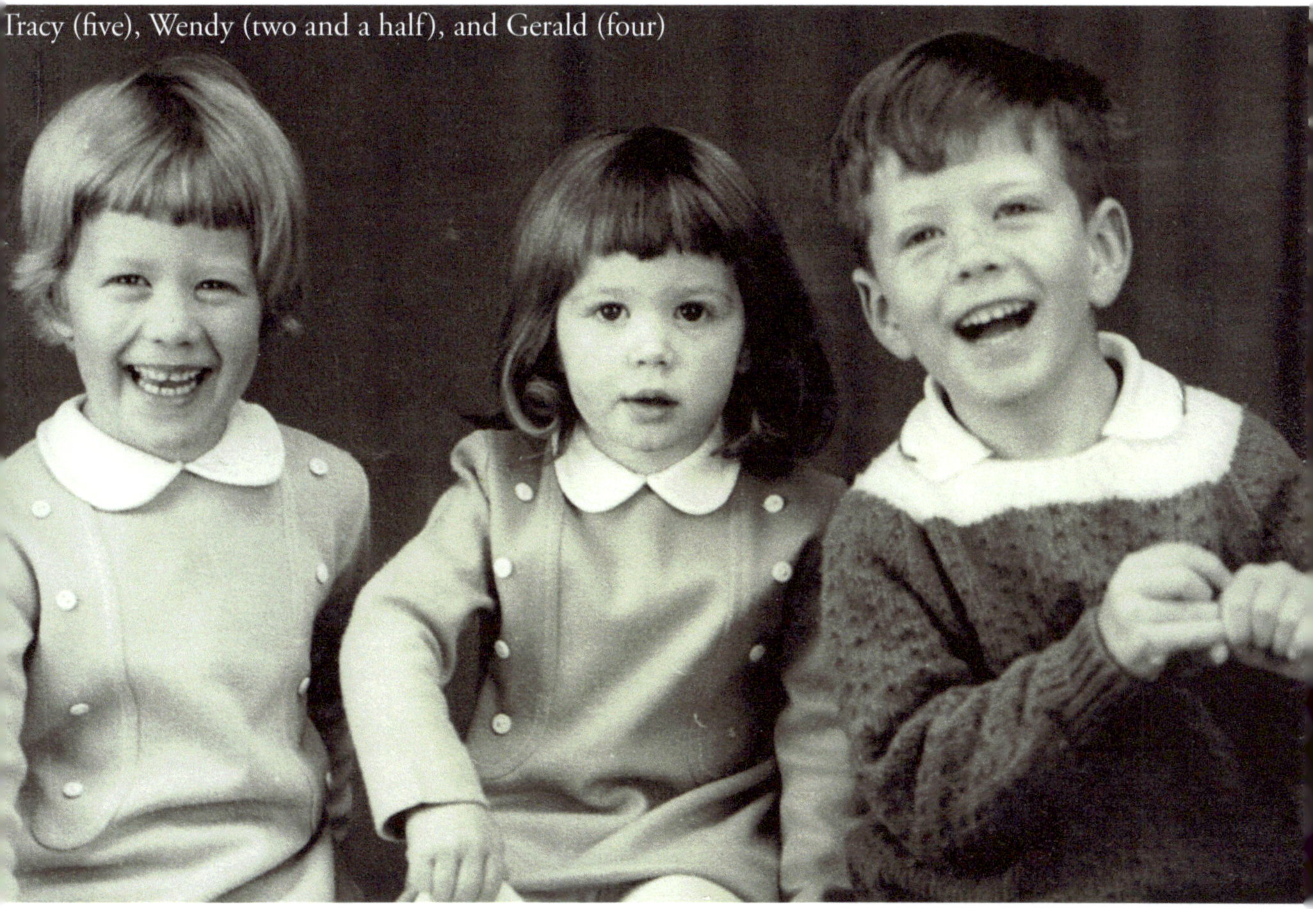

Tracy (five), Wendy (two and a half), and Gerald (four)

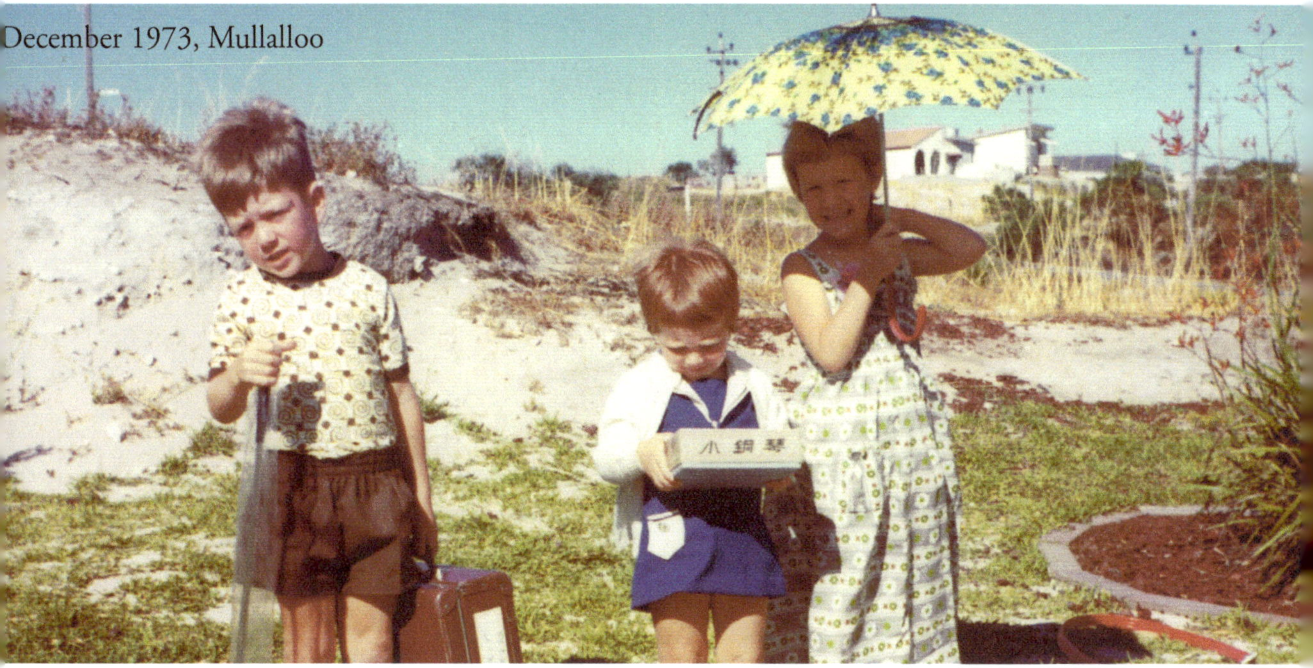

December 1973, Mullalloo

AUSTRALIA

We had not decided where in Australia we would settle and thought, 'We get off the ship in Fremantle and have a look around. If we don't like it, we can go to Melbourne or Sydney.'

Brian's cousin Graham Ledgerwood had migrated to Perth a few years ago with his wife, Mavis. They had organised for us to stay at Beatty Lodge for the first few days. After we arrived, they told us they had friends in Mullaloo, who were going to Adelaide for a month and we could stay in their house if we wanted. This was great! It gave us time to look around and see if we liked Perth enough to stay. We did! And Brian started to look for a job. This did not take long. Mavis and Graham were an excellent source of information in those first few weeks. They also had three children, and Mavis was great with the children. She looked after them sometimes, and the children loved it there. I never forget that she let the children paint on her sliding door, which the kids loved.

We each had a boy, and two girls and Peter and Gerald got on very well. The girls also played nicely together. The job Brian found was in Brunswick

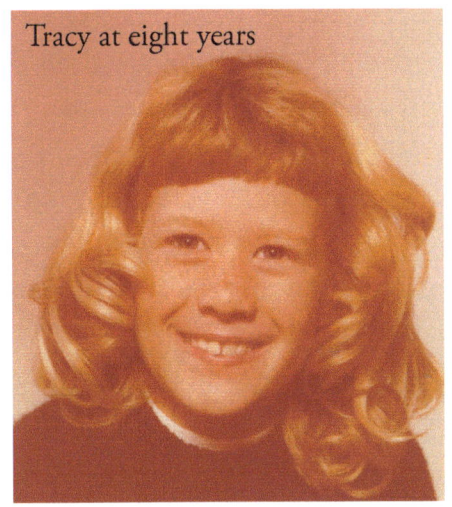
Tracy at eight years

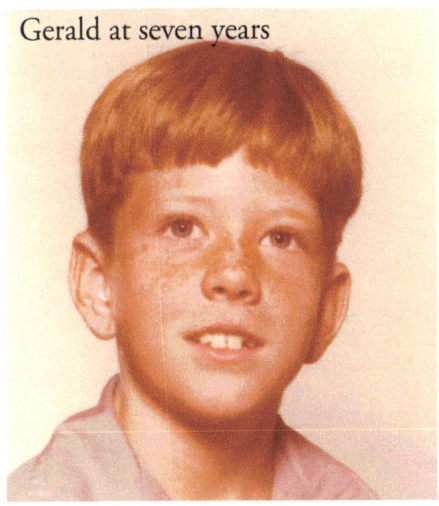
Gerald at seven years

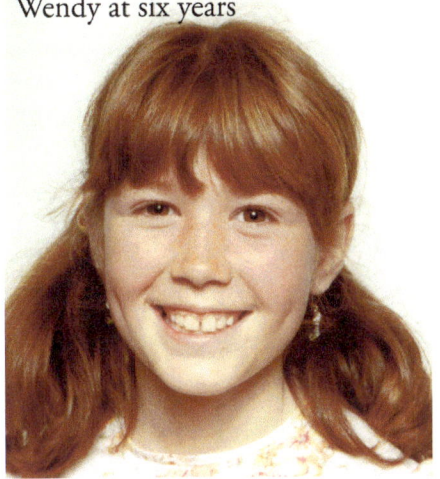
Wendy at six years

Junction, a small town between Harvey and Bunbury. I found a job in Harvey Hospital, working weekend evenings from 3 pm until 11 pm which was perfect as Brian was then home to look after the children.

We enjoyed living in the country, and Brian loved to travel around the South West and enjoyed getting to know the farmers whom he again tried to convince to raise the calves on Denkavit milk powder instead of on fresh milk

Having been accustomed to having servants in South Africa the seven years we lived there, I found it at first a challenge to do all the housework and looking after the children and working the weekends, but I got used to it pretty quickly. After all, I did grow up in a large family in Holland. It had been nice in South Africa to come home from work and find the house spotless, the washing and ironing done. But we found the people in Brunswick very friendly, and we settled in quickly. I joined the County Women's Association and the Red Cross and soon made some friends. Brian joined the bowling club.

I was very pleasantly surprised that I was paid so well. I earned the same doing only two shifts as I had from working full time in Paarl, hurrah for penalty rates! Never before had I had extra pay for working weekends!

I sometimes went with Brian on his country trips and we would take Wendy too. Our neighbour Gloria would look after Tracy and Gerald after school on such occasions, or I would arrange with their friend's mums to pick them up. They both had made friends by now.

I really wanted the children to keep up their Afrikaans and thought, 'if we speak Afrikaans at dinner and French at bath time they will be multilingual like me.' Alas, that did not work. They refused and kept telling me, "mum don't talk so funny! People here don't talk like that; we don't want to speak like that". There was nothing I could do about it, and so, when my mum came to visit, they could not understand her, which was a shame as my mum only speaks Dutch. However, they seemed to get along very well as my mum taught them a few easy card games. She even gave them some money, so they played for money! Which they thought was great! I have very happy memories of our time in Brunswick Junction and liked the South West very much. Brian's mum also came to visit while we lived there.

Brian bought a boat as we were close to Australind where we could launch it, but that was not a great success. The children were too small to enjoy it, and we sold it again and bought a caravan. This was a much better investment as we had many holidays over the next years in the caravan. We travelled all over the state. The children saw a lot of the country that way as it was affordable.

Petrol was cheap, and the parks did not charge much. As we always cooked our own meals, that did not cost more than eating at home. We sold it for $3,000 after many years, which was what it had cost us new! It was probably the best investment of our whole lives, as we did make some big mistakes along the way.

What is it with us? Again, after two and a half years Brian was transferred to Perth to head the vegetable department at Peters. And again, we moved, the story of our lives. The house we had lived in Brunswick was rented, so now we had to buy a house in Perth.

Tuart Hill seemed a reasonably priced suburb so we bought a modest three-bedroom house near the Primary school. I had started to look for a suitable job when I saw an ad in the paper. Myers was looking for nurses to do ear piercing on Friday and Saturday. So I had to find someone to look after Wendy, who was at kindy now and that is how I found Josephine, who had a son the same age, called Paul. She became an excellent friend. Josephine and Angie Di Vita had three boys, and we often went ten pin bowling with our families.

Wendy and Paul went to kindy in the morning and Josephine would pick them up and look after them until I came home. Brian would be looking after the children on Saturday while I was ear piercing at Myers. This was my first job in Perth. My second job was in a nursing home in Tuart Hill. I would work the weekend evening shift from 3 pm - 11 pm.

I also worked for a while as a sales representative for a company selling medical equipment to nursing homes and hospitals. That was not easy as there was a lot of competition from bigger companies. I used to feel really bad if I came back to the office without an order. I did sell once a few incubators to King Edward Hospital! Still, selling is not my forte, and after four months I applied to Silver Chain and got a job with them which I enjoyed. I had also applied to school health at the same time, and when they contacted me a few months later, I accepted a job at Mirrabooka High School. I would get the school holidays off, so I would be home for the children.

So, life was comfortable. We were paying the mortgage and managing some lovely holidays with the family and a 16 ft. York caravan.

Brian's mum came to visit and then my mum came again.

We decided to hire a second caravan and take my mum to Denmark. We each drove a trailer and mum had her own van, so she had some privacy. The caravan park was at Ocean Beach and mum so enjoyed herself.

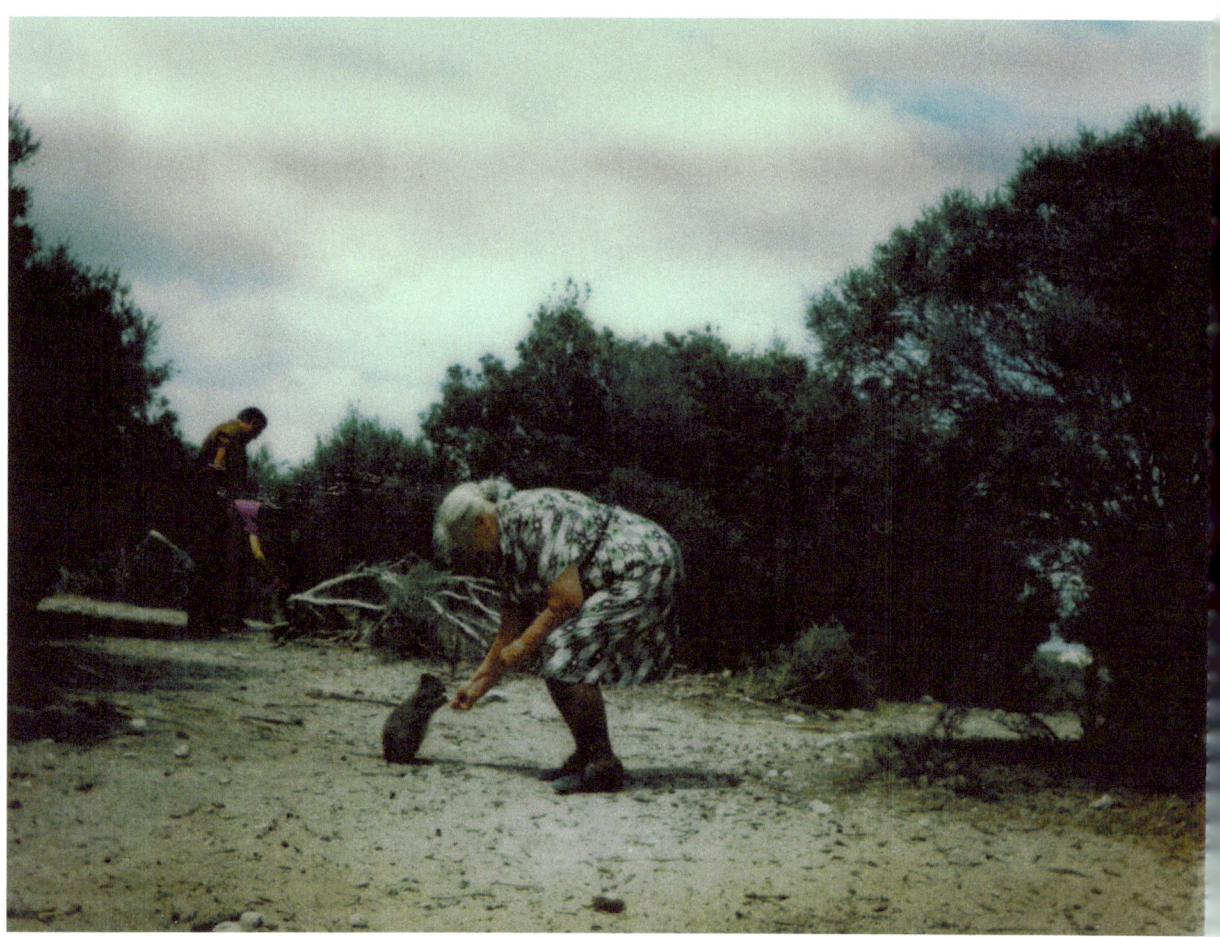

My mother at Rottnest, feeding a quokka

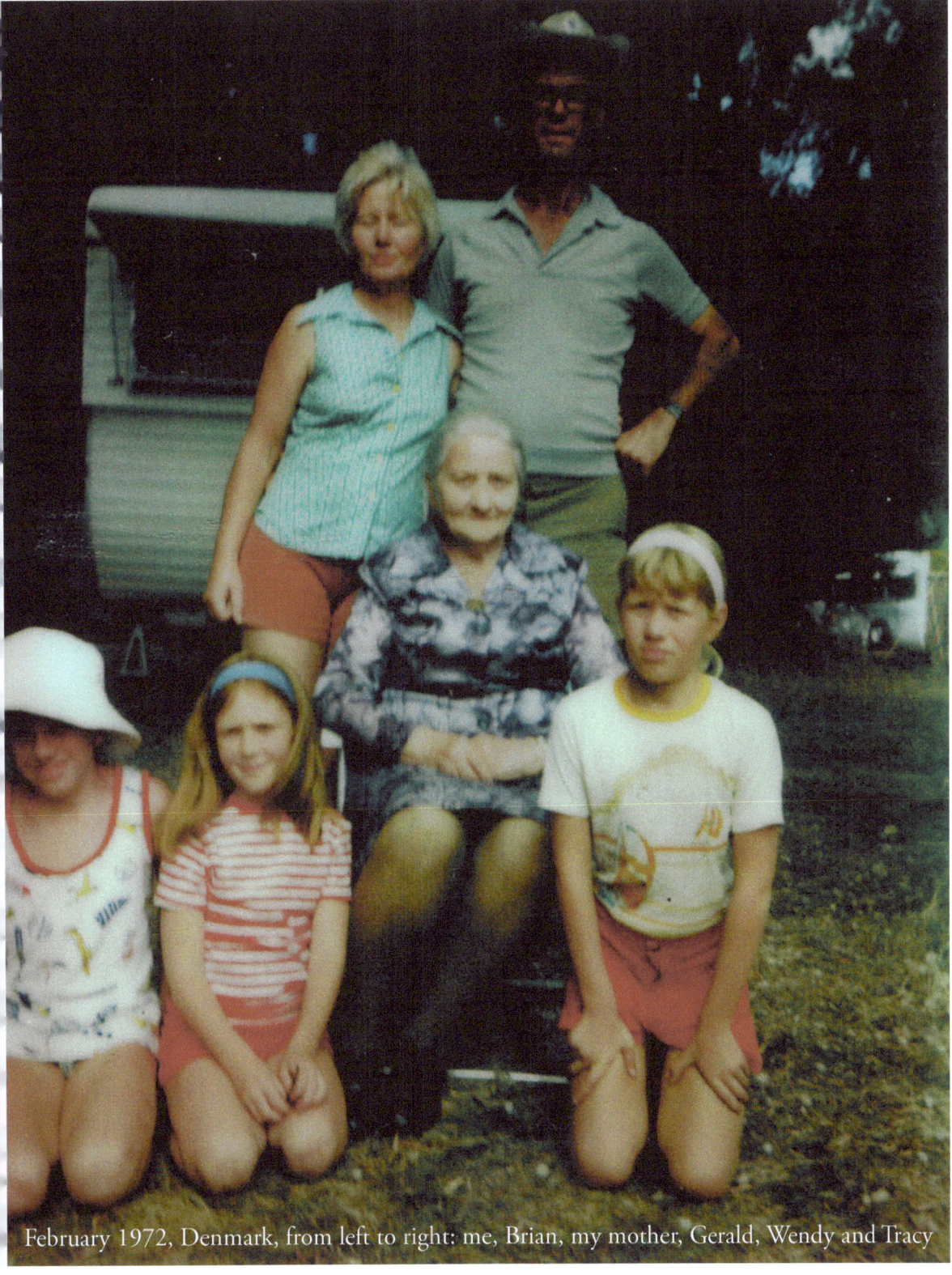

February 1972, Denmark, from left to right: me, Brian, my mother, Gerald, Wendy and Tracy

Unfortunately, things did not stay this way. Brian was working for Peters, and the new management decided that they wanted younger staff, so most people over forty-five got retrenched with only one month notice.

Brian soon found another job, but it was in Kununurra, in the very North of Western Australia, 3000 kilometres from Perth. We had been there on holidays and our cousins Graham and Mavis had in fact moved there a year ago, so we were quite excited. I was going to resign from my job at Mirrabooka but was told, "no don't resign, there may be a chance of a job in Kununurra, as there is not a school nurse there." The school did not have a medical centre, but they organised a small 13 foot caravan that I would be able to use. At least it would have air conditioning!

Brian was working for the Coop. Selling the crops from the farms, so we got to know some of the farmers. The climate was tropical, so very hot, apart from June and July. I found the heat much more difficult to take than in New Guinea as I was now forty-seven, and besides having a job, having a husband and family to care for.

The high school at that time only went to year ten, so as our eldest daughter Tracy was due to start year eleven we left Kununurra to go back to Perth as we did not want to send the children away to boarding school.

We did enjoy our two and a half years in Kununurra and saw a lot of the Kimberley and part of the Northern Territory in that time. Every holiday we would travel with the caravan. Several times to Darwin and Ayers Rock (now Uluru) and once Brian's sister and her family met us in Cairns in Queensland, and we spent a pleasant week with them exploring the Great Barrier Reef and part of Queensland.

It was at this time that I started to notice a slight change in Brian. A bit of drooling on his pillow at night, a small change in his facial expression, and then he started to drag his left foot. I suspected Parkinson's disease. Knowing there is no cure I decided not to alarm him and wait until we were back in Perth to suggest a visit to the GP who as I had expected, made an appointment to see a neurologist. He was diagnosed with Parkinson's disease. He only was forty-eight years old!

At this point, I must tell you that Brian had an abhorrence of any

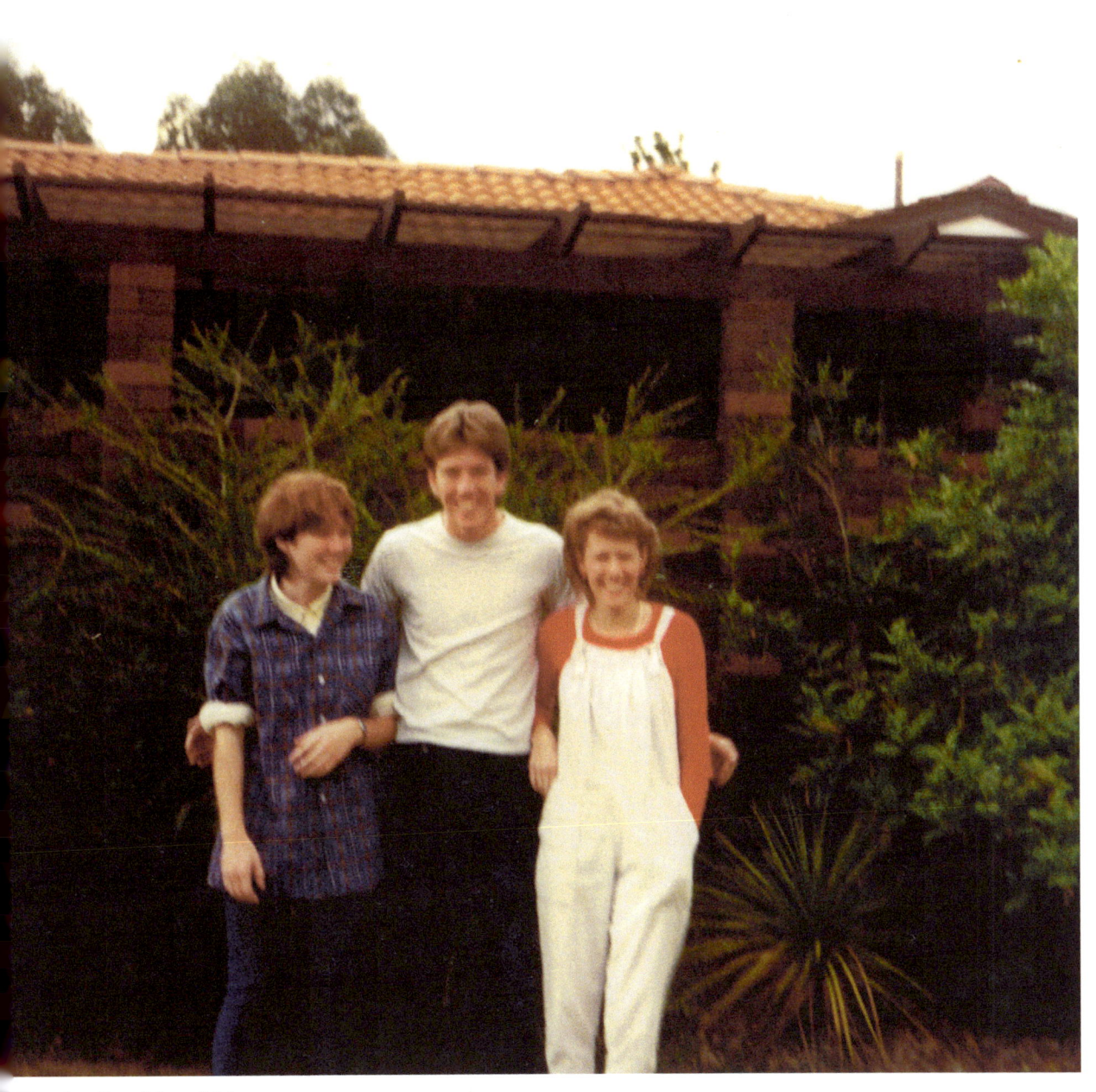
Wendy, Gerald and Tracy

disability. If we went for a walk and he saw someone with, for example, cerebral palsy, he would turn around and walk another route. If there were a television program showing anything medical, he would get upset and turn the television off. So how would he cope with this diagnosis? Well, he was started on a low dose of levodopa which controlled his early symptoms, and he did not want to know what the future was going to bring.

Back in Perth he soon found work in sales of a different kind, eventually selling caravans which he enjoyed. I got a transfer to Duncraig high school. I suggested to Brian to join the Parkinson's Association, but he declined. He enjoyed playing bowls and golf and lived in blessed ignorance of what lay ahead for almost ten years. His left foot was dragging much worse now, and he used to wear a pair of shoes out every three months. His medication had to be regularly increased, so he started to display signs of dyskinesia, which means he had these involuntary movements of arms and head caused by the levodopa. Brian preferred to have dyskinesia and be able to walk and move, whereas some patients prefer not to take so much levodopa, with the result that they cannot move freely, but that is their choice.

After some years Brian was ready to accept his diagnosis, and we became members of the Parkinson's Association. And I may say very active members! We did a lot of fundraising! We made lots of jams, pickled onions, dried tomatoes, figs etc. Which we sold at a stall in front of Woolworths in Armadale and the proceeds were donated to the Parkinson's Disease Association (PDA). We also sold hundreds of raffle tickets at different locations.

To me, it was amazing to see the gradual change in Brian. He now wanted to learn all he could about his condition and was willing to share his experiences. We started a support group in Armadale, and we met once a month with other people with Parkinson's disease (PD) and their partners. We shared and learned from each other. We attended the seminars that the Association put on regularly and were asked if we would like to become members of the speakers' group.

This was before we had any specialist nurses. It was long felt, that when a person with PD was admitted to hospital or nursing home, the staff knew very little about PD, so we became educators. We would visit hospitals and nursing homes, who had patients with PD and talk to the staff.

I would first do an introductory talk about PD, and then Brian would answer any questions. We also regularly were invited to talk to physiotherapy and speech therapy students and student nurses. Meeting a patient with PD and a carer made it much more memorable for the students. We always got very positive feedback. Once Brian lost his speech, he would answer the questions on his light writer (a computer where he could type, and it would speak for him). We travelled to Albany and Bunbury and Geraldton and to see Brian happily sharing his experiences never ceased to amaze me.

We now have specialist nurses who apart from visiting patients at home and liaising with doctors and nurses, also have taken over the role the speakers' group used to fill, such as giving talks to students. I still feel that it made more impact on the students, to meet a patient and partner and felt sorry to see the speakers' group ending.

In 1996 we heard about a new development in the treatment of PD. It was found that by making a small incision in the pallidus of the brain, the severe dyskinesia would greatly improve. Brian was a suitable candidate for this operation. He was very dyskinesic and only sixty-six years old.

We were warned of the risks, and I was not in favour of him having the pallidotomy. But as it was his body it was his choice, being the eternal optimist he was, he said: if ninety percent of patients improve then I will not belong to the ten percent who do not, so I want to have the operation. And so he did. He was the sixth patient in Perth to have the procedure. As soon as I saw him after the surgery, I knew there was something wrong. He could not speak or swallow. When I asked the surgeon about this, he said that that was quite normal, and it would improve after a few days. Well, it never did.

Brian had had a stroke, and nobody ever admitted to it. My suspicion was at last confirmed after Brian's death. I asked to read the post-mortem report which I was granted. The operation had caused massive bleeding in the brain!

Life was now getting much harder for Brian, but he never complained. He kept playing bowls for another year and golf with the help of a buggy for as long as he could hit the ball.

He used to say, "I concentrate on what I still can do and not on what I can't do." He had an incredibly positive attitude.

This was also the time that our children had their children and Brian got to enjoy all his grandchildren apart from the last one, Breanna (Wendy's fifth child), who was born after Brian died.

In these last years, we still did some travelling which we both enjoyed.

I forgot to mention that Brian insisted on buying the caravan business where he used to work as a salesman. His boss went to England saying he had emphysema and wanted to sell. A colleague and Brian went into partnership and bought the business. The worst decision ever made. I was very much against it, but Brian could be very persuasive, and at last, I agreed.

After a few months, his boss came back from England and opened another yard six kilometres up the road. He let all his customers know he was back and you can guess the rest.

We were losing money every week. We lost our home and had to start renting. Fortunately, I was still working, but this was a tough time. Brian could not work anymore. The owner of our rental had gone to the country for two years, but wanted to come back after six months! I felt, I can't cope with having to move all the time, so I went to the bank to see if I could get a loan on my super, and yes, I could. But, paying interest only, which was then thirteen percent! Now we had to find a house for no more than my super was going to be and luckily, we did. We found a free standing unit for $55,000 and close to the centre of Armadale. I was working in school health in the Armadale district, so this was very convenient.

We still managed to do a bit of travelling and spent a week in Bali. I had expected Bali to remind me of New Guinea but was very disappointed. Instead it was full of tourists and everywhere we went we were hassled by hawkers.

We did see a lot of the island, and as taxis were cheap, we travelled all over. Nothing reminded me of New Guinea apart from the climate and the language.

We also did a home exchange with a family in Adelaide and spent a month there and also with a family in Melbourne from where we went over to Tasmania which we both very much enjoyed. We also exchanged cars, so these holidays did only cost us the trip there. We took the bus to Adelaide and flew to Melbourne.

We also managed a trip to New Zealand which was particularly nice for Brian, as one of his best mates from South Africa had moved to Auckland, and we could visit them there. We particularly enjoyed the train journey from Christchurch to the West Coast. The scenery is spectacular! We were on a coach tour of both islands.

In 1999 when I could see Brian's condition was deteriorating rapidly, I asked him where he would like to go for one last holiday? He was by now fed entirely by PEG (a tube straight into his stomach) as he could not swallow at all anymore. He could not speak and communicated only with the help of his light writer. He was drooling excessively as he was producing a lot of saliva which he could not swallow. Brian had been looking at brochures, and his choice totally surprised me. He pointed at a camping holiday to the centre of Australia with Casey's, an Australian company based in Perth. I said, "but Brian, that is a camping trip! You have to sleep in a tent!". "I can do it," he insisted. "Yes, but I don't know if the company will take us. We would need a lot of extra space for all your cans and things."

Anyway, I rang Brian Casey and explained our situation. This was Brian's last wish, and as I was a nurse I would look after him, but we would need to take ninety cans of food and extra clothes amongst other things. His answer was, "bring your husband to the depot, so I can see if he can get in and out of the coach and if he can get up from the stretcher." So, we did, and this shows the kind of company Casey's is. After meeting Brian, he said, "as long as you take all responsibility, we will take him! No problem." Well, Brian was delighted!

The first day on the coach the other passengers must have wondered what is this man doing on a trip like this? But we had this lovely girl Larissa who was the tour guide and cook, and she asked me if I would take the microphone and explain what was wrong with Brian, which was a brilliant idea. So, I explained that Brian had advanced Parkinson's disease and could only communicate with his light writer. He could not swallow and drooled a lot. I would be feeding him through the PEG. At mealtimes, we would sit apart, so as to not make anybody uncomfortable. And in the various caravan camps I would come into the men's bathroom as Brian needed help, but not to be embarrassed as I was a nurse. I talked about how his mind was not affected, and if anybody would like to, he would very much enjoy some company and a chat or a joke.

Well, that trip turned out to be something extraordinary! Everybody was so understanding and friendly that it often brought tears to my eyes. Brian was in his element! He loved it when someone came over to chat with him. It is customary on these camping trips that everyone helps with the preparation of the food and the washing up, setting up of the tents and packing away of equipment. As I had a full-time job showering and toileting Brian, getting him dressed and undressed, and feeding him, I did not always have time to help with the chores, but always someone would say, "don't worry Cathy, I will do your share."

Although it was arduous work for me, I am so glad Brian got to enjoy this last holiday to Uluru and Alice Springs. When we got to Kings Canyon, Larissa asked me if I wanted to do the walk of three hours along the top of the canyon. I said I would love to, but I can't leave Brian. She said, "you go and I will look after Brian."

I had a lovely walk, and Brian enjoyed helping Larissa preparing the evening meal. He was a good cook, even if he could not eat anymore.

Larissa told me afterwards that she always had had "a thing" about people with disabilities, but that Brian had helped her to get over it.

She kept teasing Brian that he had to boogie with her in Alice Springs! And true to her word, she got him onto the dance floor and even took his hankie out of his pocket, to wipe his drooling mouth as if that was the most normal thing to do.

I tell you, there was not a dry eye in the pub that night. They talked about golf and Larissa said that on her next break she wanted to have a game of golf with him and she did! What a wonderful girl. It gave Brian such pleasure to be treated like a normal person.

There was an opportunity to have a hot air balloon ride in Alice Springs. Brian wanted to do it. As he could not climb into the basket, they held the basket on its side so he could slide in. He was lying on his back for half an hour before they set the basket upright. I could not believe how he did it, but we both enjoyed the flight over the desert.

I rang Larissa a few days before Brian died and she came to our home to say goodbye to Brian. I will never forget her.

Brian died on the 10th of September 2000 aged 68.

As the last six months had been very hard for both of us, it was actually a relief when he left us. I was so tired and slept for days after the funeral.

As none of Brian's family had been here for the funeral, his brother Cecil invited me in January 2001 to come over as they wanted to organise a memorial for Brian in Cape Town for the family and his old friends. His sister Ethel and her husband Jim came over from England, and we all stayed at Cecil and Lesley's, which was really nice. The tape of the funeral was played, and then everyone talked about how they remembered Brian. As his mum could not be there, I travelled to Utrecht afterwards to spend some time with her as her health was deteriorating. She lived on the farm with Una and Neil.

BEING A WIDOW

After a long rest, I started to think, what now? I am sixty-seven and in good health, what would I really like to do from here on? I have always loved travelling, but we did not have any savings left. As I owned my home and car and did not have any debt, I could comfortably live on the age pension, but if I wanted to travel, I needed more. Maybe I could go back to work, but my nursing registration had expired, as I had not expected ever to nurse again.

I rang the nurses' board and asked what my options were. I was told my age was not a barrier, but I had to do a re-registration course of six weeks theory and six weeks practice. They told me I was in luck as there was a course starting in Fremantle next week. I rang, and there was a vacancy, so I started the course.

I had been hospital trained in Holland in the early fifties, and this course was based on the present university course. I had never in my life done an assignment, and English not being my first language, I struggled with the wording. I had to rewrite every assignment. I was the eldest in the class, and not everyone passed, but I did! So, I was quite proud of myself.

I had my registration back and found a job at a new nursing home in Kelmscott. In Australia one cannot receive the age pension while working, so I had to go off the pension, which is fair enough.

I started saving and could travel again.

BORNEO

My first trip after Brian's death was to Borneo. This trip included a five-day trek (the head-hunter's trail) which did remind me a lot of New Guinea. We were a small group of seven people with a guide, and the trip also included climbing Mt. Kinabalu, which is a two-day climb with a stop at Laban Ratu overnight. Then the next morning a very early rise at 2 am to trek to the top to see the sunrise.

Unfortunately, I did not make it to the top as just before reaching Laban Ratu I fell over some big rocks and broke some ribs. I had hired a porter to carry my backpack, and this young girl found me a second stick, so I managed to reach our overnight stop. The rest of the group was already there, and the guide suggested I bind myself up with a sarong which helped and I had enough Panadol with me for the pain. However, I decided not to join the group for the climb to the summit, but instead leave at 6 am for the descent. I did not carry anything, and with the help of two sticks, I managed quite well. I arrived down the mountain at the same time as the rest of the group and enjoyed the rest of the tour as it did not include any more walking. We had a lovely day on the Kinabatangan river seeing proboscis monkeys and some beautiful birds. When we stopped for lunch I could not see where we would eat, but out of the bush came these people with all sort of dishes with delicious food. It was quite amazing. Our overnight stop was a lovely place in the jungle.

All in all, a delightful trip.

RETURNING TO WORK

I worked at the nursing home in Kelmscott for about six months when I saw an advert for a nursing post in Tjuntjuntjara, an Aboriginal settlement in the Great Victoria Desert. I applied and was invited to come for an interview. My flight was paid for. I had to fly to Kalgoorlie with Qantas and then further with a small plane from the flying doctor's service. There was another young couple on board of the plane, and they told me they were also going for an interview. They were both nurses too.

The interview went well. The next day I got a phone call when they told me, as they needed two nurses they had chosen the couple. As the couple would like their leave together, was I interested in working as a reliever?

As you get quite a lot of leave in those jobs, that would mean I would go out there every three months for a month. Perfect! I accepted, and I would have to let Centrelink know every time I left to go off the pension, and when I came back so that I would get the pension back again.

I saved enough while I was working as there was nothing to spend money on. All I paid for was rent and food. I enjoyed the work. The clinic was open from 7:30 am to 12 pm and 2 to 5 pm. After that, I was on call in case of emergencies. The flying doctor visited once a fortnight and would come out anytime in case of an emergency. The nurses' home was next to the clinic.

There was a small shop that sold fresh food and veggies. There were a few other non-indigenous people, for example, the teachers. I became friendly with them, and we sometimes shared a meal.

Tuntjuntjara is a dry community which means there is no alcohol allowed. I was very pleased about that. From my observations, many indigenous Australian's don't have good drinking habits. Once they start drinking they find it difficult stop. When drunk they become aggressive and abusive and look for a fight; I believe, purely a result of alcohol being an introduced product that they have not grown accustomed to over generations in the same way as Eurasian people. So, I was pleased that the elders in the community had decided on a dry community.

There would typically be about 300 people having their home here, but this could vary a lot. Whenever there was a funeral or a wedding, many people from miles away would come, so the population could quickly grow to 400 or more. Equally, the town would almost empty if there was a funeral or wedding elsewhere. This would cause a lot of headache for the medical staff.

Each person on medication would be given a box with their script to last a week. They often would forget to take theirs with them or ask for extra. The same happened with people coming from other communities. We then had to ring the nurse in those places to find out what medication the person was on and then give them enough to make it back home. Diabetes was very prevalent, and they would often forget their insulin syringe.

The medical care the people in these remote areas get is excellent; twenty-four hour access to a nurse and a doctor's visit once a fortnight. In case of an emergency a flying doctor on call! And everything is totally free! They pay no fee for medicine or dental care. Even their dogs get vaccinated free of charge, a vet comes out every six months.

There is only paid work available for a few people. A few people work in the office, and a few prepare 'meals on wheels' for the elderly. They get paid. A few people collect the rubbish and burn it and the rest of the people get a pension.

Many of the young people prefer to live in the city and leave the community. If they want to study or do an apprenticeship, they get a lot of support. Though I've seen many, who have a 'chip on their shoulder' and expect too much without any effort.

I enjoyed the experience and found most people friendly and easy to get on with.

Mark and Leo, who I had been relieving, had gotten married and wanted to return to Melbourne. As I had turned seventy by now, I decided to call it a day as well, as the work was getting a bit much. I had been doing the job of two nurses and started to feel my age. I had a bit of savings now so where to next? I had been doing some research and found an interesting tour with World Expeditions to Vietnam. It was 2003.

VIETNAM

The tour started in Saigon but did not include the Mekong Delta which I wanted to see. So, I booked a few extra days before the tour to visit the Mekong Delta. I had a private tour with a driver and a guide and was treated like a princess. The meals were fantastic! I would have preferred to eat with the driver and the guide, but that did not seem customary. I was served these large platters with beautifully cut out vegetables and fruit in the shape of people or boats. They looked like works of art! It was far too much for one person. So as not to waste the leftovers, I asked for an extra plate and dished myself up what I could eat, hoping the family would have a bit of a feast as well. I am sure they don't eat like that themselves normally.

    I was amazed by the size of the Delta. So many tributaries of the Mekong came out of all directions to eventually run out into the China Sea. So many people live on boats, making a living from fishing or trading fruit or vegetables, some from their farms, others buying and selling. A hive of activity! The boats are not big, but people manage to eat, sleep, cook and trade their wares. While bringing up their family. This is their home!

After a few days, we were back in Saigon and met with our group. I shared a room with a very nice forty-year-old lady from Melbourne. She was a dancer and great fun. In spite of our age difference we got on ever so well and had lots of laughs. We first travelled to Dalat up in the mountains which was a lot cooler than Saigon. There is a noticeable French influence in Vietnam due to the 300 years of French occupation which is visible in the architecture, the wide boulevards and also in the food. Especially in the bread and pastries. I learned a bit about the history, but am no expert, so won't go into that.

The Vietnamese people have suffered terribly over the centuries, not least during the last Vietnam War. I was touched by their attitude towards tourists French and Americans alike. They treated all with respect saying, "we can never forget, but we can forgive and try to look forward to the future as an independent nation at last." Wow!

We saw a lot of poverty. Many people with missing limbs due to the many landmines all over the countryside. We did all our travel on land by small coach or train. When we got to Hoi An some of us had some clothes made as there are some excellent tailors and the materials are beautiful. You choose the material and the suit or dress you want. You get measured, and twelve hours later the completed outfit is delivered to your hotel. I had a fully lined pantsuit made with two silk blouses to go with.

We travelled to Hue and many other places ending up in Hanoi from where we went to Haloing Bay where we spent a night on a houseboat. As we swam off the houseboat one of our group, (a Canadian with an artificial leg), had a lot of interest from the Vietnamese as so many of them have missing limbs but have never seen any artificial limbs. All in all, this had been a fascinating and enjoyable tour.

My third brother Ben had been diagnosed with pancreatic cancer. I wanted to go and see him and asked him if he would like me to come over soon or rather wait until later when he might need some nursing care. He said, "come now while I am still able to go for short walks and sit out in the garden." So, I booked and went to The Hague where Ben lived with his partner Netty. My brother Fons came over from Canada as well, and so we spent some quality time with Ben and the family. The weather was perfect all the time we were there so that we could enjoy the garden and some short walks. I even managed a quick trip to Paris to see my good friend Els.

Three months later Ben rang me and asked if I could come to help nurse him as it was getting too much for Netty and he did not want to go to a hospice. He paid my fare, and I went right away. Ben was in a bad way. He had lost so much weight and was very jaundiced. He had a huge ascites (stomach full of fluid, which had to be drained regularly). He wanted to receive the Last Rites, being a devout Catholic, but we had a lot of trouble finding a priest. Eventually, we found that Cor Nieuwenhuizen, an old friend of the family, was able to come on Sunday when all the family could attend.

It was amazing to see how Ben was absolutely glowing. He was so ready to die! He passed away peacefully in his sleep in the early morning of the 10th of September 2003. I felt privileged to have helped nurse him in the last week of his life.

BEING A CARER

In 2004 I was asked by the Parkinson's specialist nurse Janet if I would be interested in looking after a patient with PD, who lived on her own and did not want to go into a nursing home. She needed a carer for the weekends from Friday night until Monday morning. I agreed to meet her and found her to be a very lovely eighty-year-old lady, so every weekend I would drive to Nedlands where she lived and spend the weekend looking after her. During the week she had other carers.

I would ask her what she would like to do. On Saturdays, she usually wanted to go out. Sometimes to Kings Park, where we would have lunch at the Zamia Cafe. Sometimes to a museum, or just for a bit of a drive or a bit of shopping. She could still walk short distances with the help of a frame.

She had done a lot of travelling in her life and loved to tell me of her journeys. We enjoyed each other's company. At night she would call out if she needed any help but most nights I got a reasonably good sleep with few interruptions. I got paid to sleep!

After about eight months the family (brother and niece, she had never married) wanted her to go into a nursing home. She did not want to go. Maybe her finances were running out as it was costly to have twenty-four hours a day home care? I don't know the reason, but she had to leave her home, and although she was well looked after in the nursing home, she was not happy.

Every time I went to visit her, I felt so sad for her. She seemed to deteriorate at a much faster rate. She had become a very dear friend. She passed away very lonely.

I looked after another patient, who lived in Cottesloe, close to the beach. A very nice man with a lovely wife who was also his carer. Now and then she needed a break, and I would look after her husband whenever she wanted me to.

I was seventy-one and fortunately in good health. I enjoyed playing golf with the Dale Golf Club on a Friday. I never improved my handicap which was always around the 30, which is very high for nine holes but I enjoyed the game and the company of so many lovely people. I was also still the support group leader of the Armadale branch of the Parkinson's Association.

CANADA

In 2005 I went on a long holiday. First to Holland to see my family and then to Canada to see my brother Fons and his wife, Nel. Fons was celebrating his seventieth birthday in May. My eldest brother Frans and his wife Truus were going too. It was lovely to meet my Canadian family! Fons and Nel have five sons and to meet them all and their children was very special.

When I booked my flight through my travel agent in Armadale, he said, "why on earth would you want to spend three weeks in Toronto? Apart from the Niagra Falls, there is nothing to see." How wrong he was!

We had an absolutely fabulous time! The days that Fons could not take us out, he had arranged for his son Stephen and his wife Yasmin to take us out. They had a young son Luke who came with us everywhere. We went every day somewhere. Starting with Toronto. We saw the tower where on the top floor there is a glass floor where you can step onto and look right down. Quite scary! We went to the museum and another day to the Zoo which is a very natural zoo. We enjoyed it very much.

Another day we went to the Niagra Falls and had a ride on the 'maid of the mist', a boat that takes you right into the spray of the falls.

We also visited the Mennonites, an Amish community that lives life with few amenities; like 100 years ago. They make everything themselves including leather objects; I bought a purse that I still use today. They grow their own vegetables, milk their own cows. Grow their own beef, make their own clothes. It was very interesting. Transport is by horse and cart. No cars or TV although they have now some computers only for limited use by certain staff.

We visited the maple museum where they explained how maple syrup is made from the sap of the maple tree. A hole is bored into the bark, only one hole a year to preserve the tree. The holes are never in a line, but always in a different spot. Instead of using a bucket to catch the sap, they now catch the sap in a tube to a container. The sap only contains 3% sugar. This is then boiled, so it evaporates until it forms a syrup which contains 60% of sugar. Hence, it is very expensive!

I think of the three weeks we spent in Toronto there were only two days we did not go anywhere. When I saw my travel agent afterwards, I told him not ever to say to any of his clients that there is not much to see in Toronto. We saw so much and thoroughly enjoyed our time there.

From Toronto, I went to Calgary where I boarded the Rocky Mountaineer train. This must be one of the world's most scenic train journeys. All travel is done during the day. The train stops at night, and one sleeps in a hotel and continues the next morning. So, you do not miss anything of the fantastic scenery. Breakfast and lunch are served on the train and dinner at the hotel in Kamloops. The food and the commentary on the train were both great! We arrived in Vancouver at 5:30 pm after two delightful days. Yes, it is expensive, but if you travel that far, you should experience this train ride!

We started our Cosmos coach trip the next day. The coach took us through the same area as the train, but the scenery was not anywhere as spectacular as the coach cannot go where the train can. On the way to Banff, we passed the 'Natural Bridge', which was very beautiful. We spent a day in Banff and another day in Jasper. On the way, we saw black bears, eagles, squirrels and elk. I have not seen a moose yet. Banff is beautiful. I walked along the Bow River to the top and took the gondola back. I must have walked four hours that day. The hotels are very nice. On the way to Jasper, we passed Lake Louise where we got an hour and a half stop. The hotel here is spectacular, but we did not stop there. This is a Cosmos tour, not A.P.T. or Scenic.

We moved on to the Colombian icefields, where we had lunch first and then a ride on the glacier which was fun. Then to the Athabasca Falls. From here to the river where we got into our boats for some rafting. Our guide had told us that we would get capes, so I did not bring my cape. Big mistake as the flimsy plastic ponchos did not have sleeves, so we all got soaked wet. And were very cold. Still it was good fun! The following day we did a cruise on Maligne Lake and spent some time on Spirit Island. We also saw the Maligne Canyon. Very beautiful! Our guide Steve told us some interesting stories, like how a mother moose saved her babies from a grizzly bear. She dunked him with her paw so many times until he drowned. The moose can dive and swim for hours as her hairs are hollow giving her great buoyancy.

We drove to Prince George where we would stay two nights, then on to Prince Rupert. I was looking forward very much to the ferry ride to Victoria Island and did enjoy that very much. There was beautiful scenery all along the coast. The Butchart Gardens in Victoria did not disappoint. I spent extra time here as the rest of the group only spent a few hours. I made my own way back to the hotel. The next day back in Vancouver and then the flight back to Perth. This was another very nice trip.

CHINA

Life was excellent, and I feel very blessed that I was able to take a trip every year and did so.

There is so much to learn and see in this beautiful world, and I never get enough of seeing new places and meeting people from different cultures. I just wished that Brian could have joined me on my travels. Every weekend I read the travel insert in the paper. 'Travel' in the Saturday paper and 'Escape' in the Sunday Times. That gave me ideas what to see next.

I had noticed that Wendy Wu organised some fascinating tours at reasonable prices. The quoted prices always included airfares and all the meals as well as accommodation and transport and entree fees to all attractions. Unfortunately, they did not offer a 'willing to share' price for solo travellers. As I would travel on my own, I had to pay an extra $1,000.

Wendy Wu advertised a tour called, 'rivers and mountains', starting in Hong Kong then to Shanghai and from there right across China. I booked to go on this trip in 2006. There were only sixteen other people on tour. I was the only solo. It was very nice to have my own room, and I always got the best room. I would have a view when others did not. One morning I woke up and watched a whole lot of hot air balloons passing by. None of the others had seen them as they did not have a room with a view. I could also wash a few things when needed and hang them without having to consider space for my roommate. So, I felt it was worth the extra I paid.

We had a nice group, and someone would always invite me to join them in the free time I am still in touch with some of them, and two couples have visited me in Perth. I usually prefer to see countryside and scenery rather than big cities and this tour was perfect.

Although I always keep a diary of each trip, I will not bore you with a day to day account of what we saw. Suffice to say that I found China a very interesting and scenically very beautiful country much to my surprise! Having a forty seat coach and only seventeen people meant that everyone could have a window seat if they so wished.

The organisation was excellent, the food and accommodation and the guides all very good. I can recommend Wendy Wu as very good value for money. I would love to go back to see more as it is such a huge country. One cannot see everything in a holiday of nineteen days.

SCANDINAVIA

In 2008 I went to Scandinavia with my cousin Mavis. We first did a Cosmos Tour through Denmark, Sweden and Norway and then a cruise with the Hurtigruten Line. They are a postal service delivering food, post, building materials, and other things to all the small towns along the coast. We chose the Nordgren which is their oldest, smallest but also the cheapest ship. As they go ashore in different places on the way North as on the way South we decided to make a return trip.

At some point the captain announced that we had to rescue a small fishing boat that had lost its engine power. I quickly went on deck to watch this. I saw a little boat in the distance, and when we got close enough, our crew shot a line, but the fisherman missed. At the third attempt he caught the line, and we pulled him along for about half an hour. The sea was quite rough. Then the coast guard came along to help him, and we could resume our journey. I enjoyed watching that!

One night when we were out on the open ocean, the sea was very rough. We had to hold ourselves on the side of our bunks so as not to fall out of bed. Suddenly a mighty crash. What was that? Neither of us was game to investigate, and the next morning we found that the only chair in our cabin had moved across and crashed into the wall. Fortunately, neither of us get seasick so we thoroughly enjoyed the cruise. The food was fabulous. Breakfast and lunch, you helped yourself to all the seafood you wanted. Herring, salmon, caviar and the like! I did not know that there is white and pink as well as black caviar! But like all good things in life, a little bit of a delicacy is special. When there is so much of it, you become blasé. We enjoyed the trip very much. After returning to Copenhagen, I went to Holland to see my family and Mavis went back to Perth.

THE GIBB RIVER ROAD AND OTHER ADVENTURES

While living in the Kimberley, I had never been on the Gibb River Road. In 2009 I saw an advertisement for a camping trip from Broome to Kununurra with a return to Broome for just over $2,000. That was really cheap, so I booked. I was now seventy-six years old and had a bit of trouble pitching a tent. I had expected there to be a few people younger than me to give me a hand, but most of us were older and the only young couple on the tour must have made up their mind that they would only help themselves because they were always the last ones to get up in the morning and never helped anyone. It was really difficult as the ground was so hard. Once we got to Kununurra, I wanted to visit the school, where I had been a school nurse some thirty years ago. When I introduced myself, they asked me if I wanted to have a tour of the school. What a difference. They are now a proper high school up to year twelve and have a beautiful art area and excellent facilities. All classrooms are brick now, so no more demountables, as in my days. It was very kind of them to give me a tour. They have a proper medical centre, but no school nurse. A nurse comes a few times a week to check vision and hearing but is not available anymore in case students feel unwell.

While we had two free days in Kununurra, I did a cruise on the Ord River and was pleasantly surprised that the person who owned that business, was a man that used to be in year seven when I was the school nurse thirty years ago, Ashleigh Cummings! When he realised who I was, he gave me a discount! The other free day I did a cruise on the Ord River Dam, which brought back lots of memories. I managed to catch up with an old friend, Frauke Boshammer, who invited me to dinner and I met up with her daughter Margret and her children. Margret and Wendy were friends, and so were Fritz and Gerald. It was really lovely to see them all.

On the trip was a very nice couple from Switzerland. I always find it amusing when people from some European countries (Denmark as well) find it so natural to swim in the nude. Most of us would wear bathers, but not them! Anyway, I enjoyed their company as their English was not very good and they were happy I could speak French. They invited me, should I ever come to Switzerland to go and see them, which I did in 2010 when Mavis and I did a tour of Switzerland and Italy. They insisted that we cancelled our hotel and stayed with them. They showed us around Geneva, where they live, and we spend a few very nice days with them.

Also in 2009, my friend Dessa wanted to do a trek in Nepal, I was happy to go with her to Nepal, but not sure about trekking. After the first day, which had been hours of climbing, I was exhausted and so was Dessa. I asked our guide what our options were as I did not think I could go on. He told us, "no problem, I will send you back with a porter, and a guide and you can stay in our camp in Pokhara until we meet you there in another four days." Dessa was very disappointed, but although she is ten years younger than me, she could not have done it. I said, "it is not a holiday if it is too hard, so let's enjoy the time in Pokhara", which we did. Dessa had a massage every day because her back was killing her. The rest of the tour was by vehicle and very interesting.

In 2010 I went to Holland again and had a lovely time. My niece and nephew had a boat and took me several days for a cruise on the waters around them. My sister took me to the Krollemuller museum which has a lot of Vincent van Gogh paintings which I enjoyed very much. I did take up oil painting in the late nineties and became a member of the Armadale Society of Artists. I used to get lessons from John Baines every Saturday afternoon, and over the few years, I produced quite a few paintings. I was not very good but enjoyed the distraction as this was at the time that looking after Brian became more difficult. I have always enjoyed art, and the years I lived in London and Paris used to be a frequent visitor to the various museums.

Last year when I was in Holland, I was pleasantly surprised to find that in my nephew's house there were two paintings of mine on the walls. I used to give them as presents when visiting family or friends.

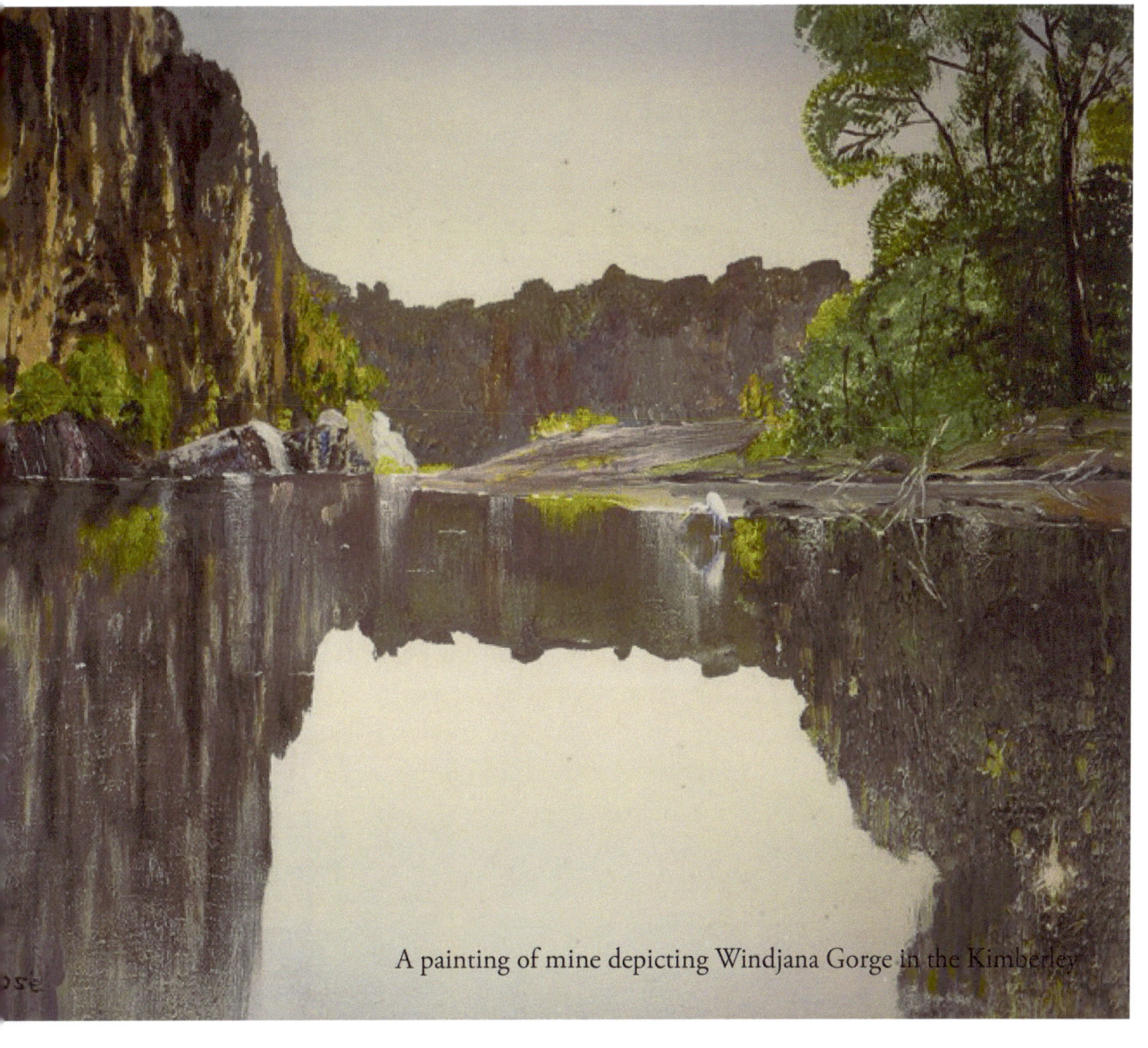

A painting of mine depicting Windjana Gorge in the Kimberley

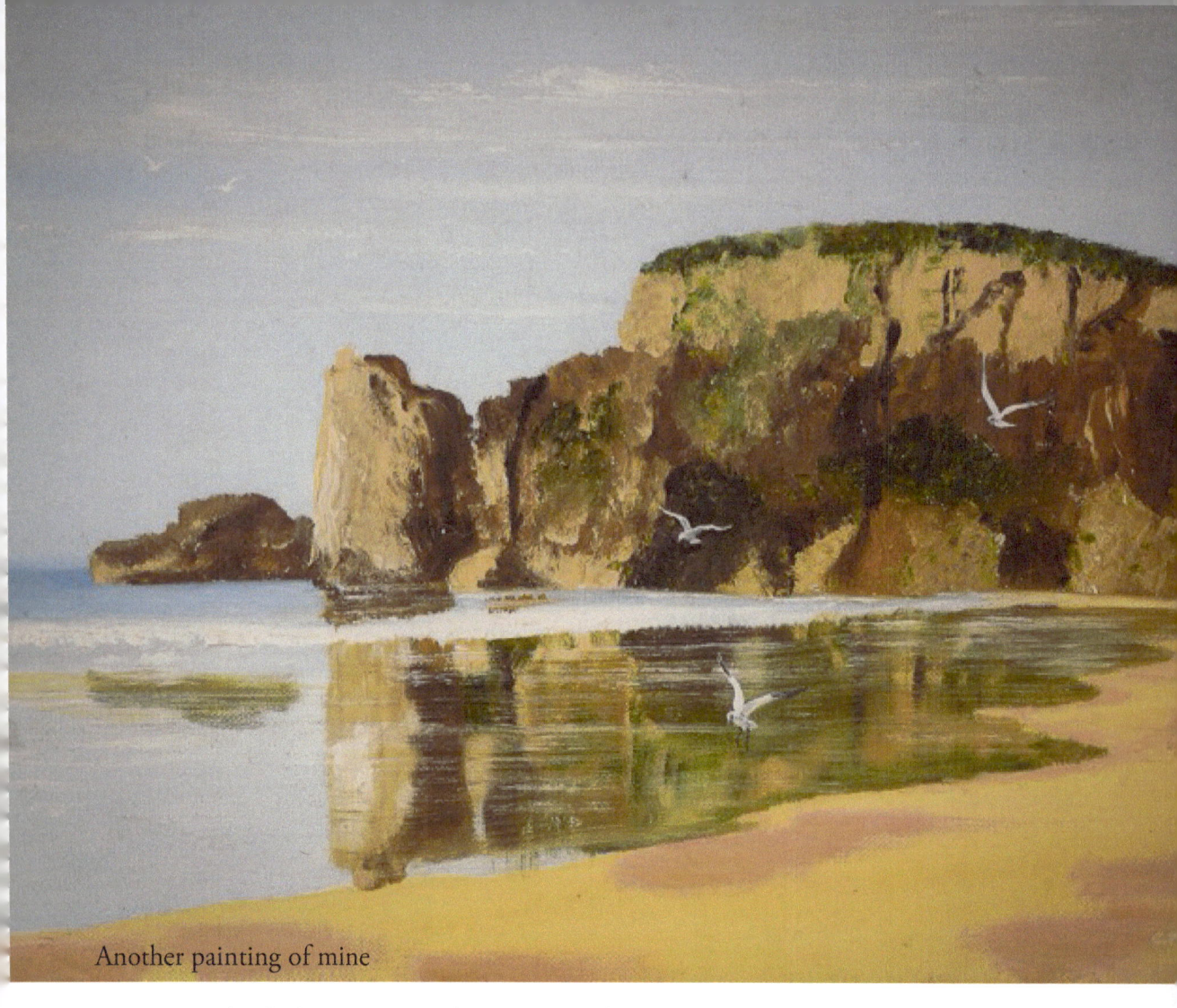
Another painting of mine

I had always wanted to see South America, so when I saw a cruise advertised from San Francisco to Buenos Aires for thirty days, I asked my sister Ans to come with me. The journey was on the Star Princess, one of the many ships of the Princess Cruise line. Unfortunately, I got sick a few times and had to be confined to my cabin, but apart from that, we had a fabulous time. We enjoyed many shore excursions and went as far south as Cape Horn. We also saw the Falkland Islands and wondered why England is so keen on them as scenically they are not worth the fuss, but of course, there is oil! However, so far England has not had the money to explore that and who knows when they will.

The cruise along the Chilean Coast was spectacular!! We thoroughly enjoyed the holiday and not least the company of my sister. As youngsters, I had always been close to my older sister Riet (who died at the age of 52 of leukaemia). So now to spend a month with my sister Ans, who is five years my junior, was beautiful, especially as she is so very different from me (a bit OCD), but here she did not have to do anything, so we spent some quality time together. We really got to know each other.

I found that I like cruising!

In 2013 my friend Bi and I went on a river cruise on the Mekong River. This was a great find as usually, river cruises are much more expensive than ocean cruises. But this was advertised at $2500, which was an excellent price for thirteen days. The reason ocean cruises are much cheaper is that the big ships can carry up to 5000 passengers, where a river cruise is always on a small vessel of no more than a few hundred.

On the river cruises, the shore excursions are mostly included, which is not the case on an ocean cruise, and that can add a fair bit to the price, but then you do not need to do all the excursions. In most places you can either stay on board, which costs nothing and there is always enough to do on board, or you can go ashore and do your own thing. Take public transport or book a cheaper tour or hire a taxi. The excursions organised by the cruise company are costly, but they show you the most exciting things to see. You always have a choice. Short or long, simple or strenuous. Always something for everyone. What we found swell about the Mekong River cruise was that we could go on an excursion in the morning and again in the late afternoon. So back on the ship for lunch and a nap as it was sweltering in the middle of the day.

In 2013 I also went on a rail trip across Java. This was organised by Bicton Travel and happens every year. The hotels were very luxurious with always a beautiful swimming pool. I seemed the only person to enjoy regular swims before breakfast. We had as a group our own carriage on the train. Very comfortable. We saw a bit of Jakarta and then went into the mountains to Bandung, which was a journey of 173 kilometres. Coffee, tea and lunch were served on board. We arrived at our hotel at 3 pm after a very relaxing trip. The next day a pleasurable drive into the mountains. Then on to the Perahu Volcano where we had a soak in a mineral bath, and after lunch, we saw a performance by children singing and playing some instruments. The next day was a long day on the train to Yogyakarta. We had our own carriage again and the day was very pleasant. We arrived in Yogyakarta at 3 pm. The bus to our hotel was waiting for us. We arrived at the hotel at 5 pm. Change and off to a local restaurant, which is a fifteen minute walk, Bessie a lady of eighty-seven years, did not feel up to the walk, so I shared a becak with her.

Meals are very cheap! I had beef rendang and a beer, which came to $7.70. I gave the waitress $10, and she was ever so pleased.

Next day we went to the Borobudur Temple. It was sweltering! The climb to the top was not easy as the steps are very high. I took it slowly. It took 100 years to build this beautiful temple. It has many levels, and each level has so many reliefs and stories. We only had an hour, and to see this temple properly, you need much more time. But as it was so hot, we were all glad to be back on the coach with air conditioning and heading off to lunch. After lunch another highlight of this tour. A trip on a 110-year-old steam train. The train climbed slowly through some admirable countryside. We went through some villages and were impressed how clean the villages looked. The train had to stop at a small stream to take on some water, and we could get off and talk to some children. An old lady of ninety came out to look at the train. She still had her eyesight and hearing and walked slowly, but independently. It was nice to have some interacting with the locals. I miss that on the more luxurious trips. All in all, this had been again a charming trip.

In May, 2014, I tried to get my friend Dessa to come with me to Croatia as that is where she comes from, but to no avail, so I went solo. I went with Insight Vacations as they had a 'willing to share' policy. If there was no one of the same sex to share with, you would get a room by yourself without having to pay the single supplement. I was in luck. Although there was another lady on her own, she had chosen to have her own room, so she paid the single supplement, and I did not. She was a bit sore about that. When she asked me if I had paid the extra and I said, "no." She said, "I would have shared with you!" I told her you must book 'willing to share', as you cannot change your mind afterwards. You take a chance, and for me, it has always worked out fine. However, I was told by one of the tour leaders that they once had a lady, who would make things so uncomfortable for her roommate that that person would then pay the extra to have her own room. And then she would have the room to herself! She managed to do that several times. That company will not take her anymore. Croatia is a wonderful country, and I found the tour very well organised. Our guide was a very nice, knowledgeable lady and we had a lovely group of people again. So this was again a very enjoyable trip.

Another trip in 2014 was an African safari! My sister in law, Elin was going to meet me in Johannesburg, and we had booked a train safari. It was called the Shongololo train. It would travel at night and have four-wheel drive vehicles on board. During the day we would go wild life spotting in different locations. We were both very much looking forward to this adventure. However, three days before I left Perth, the travel agent rang me and told me that the tour was cancelled as there were not enough passengers! Elin had also been notified and was very disappointed too. Her daughter got in touch with a travel agent in Cape Town whom she knew and asked if he could put something together for us. Starting in Johannesburg and finishing in Dar es Salaam. The safaris are usually fully booked months ahead, and we did not have much hope, but this agent knew of some new camps, which had only recently opened, and he did a fantastic job for us.

We could not have had a better time!

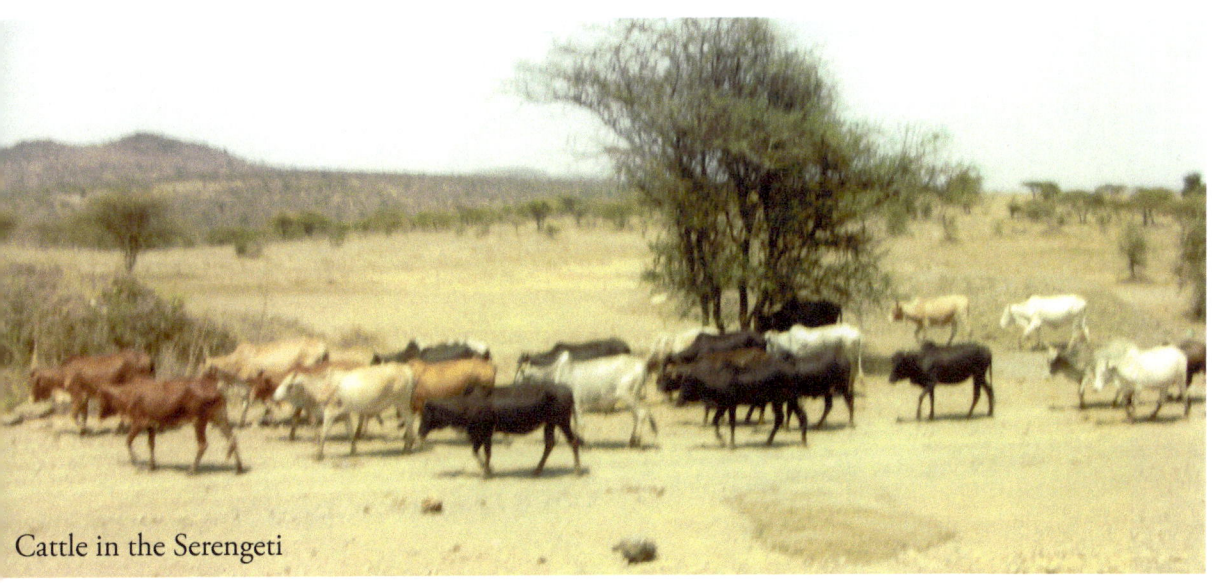

Cattle in the Serengeti

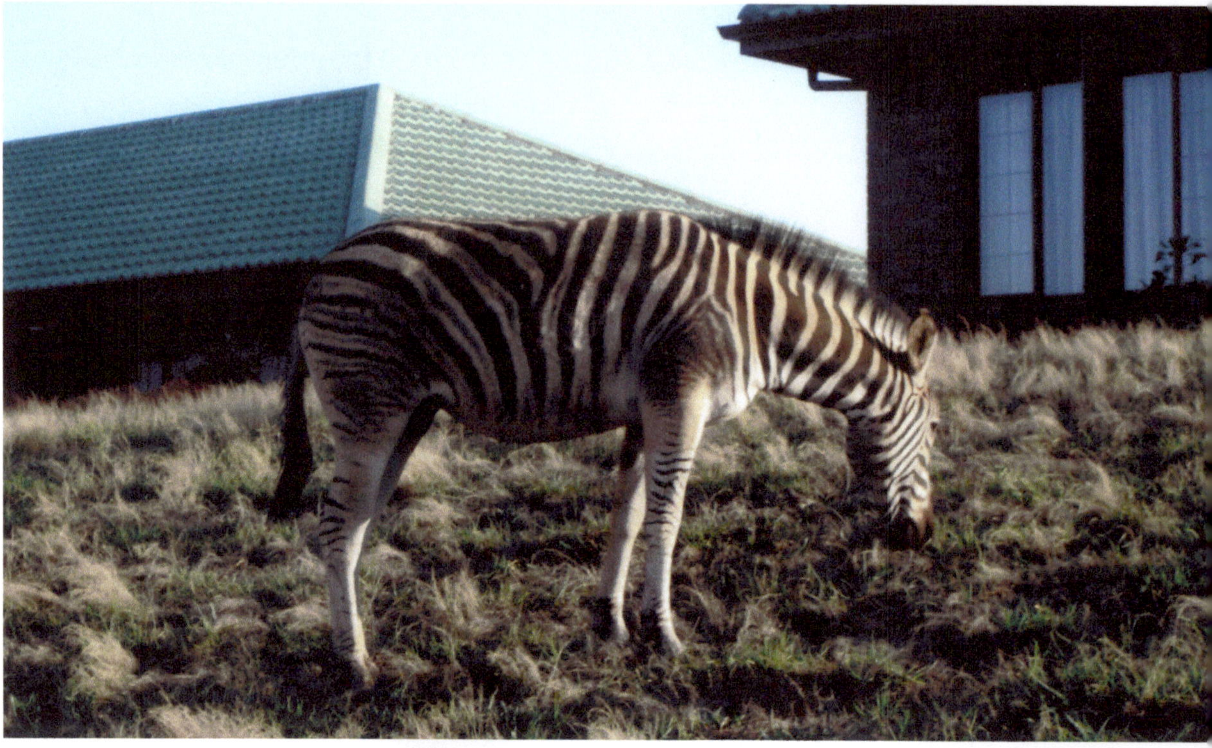

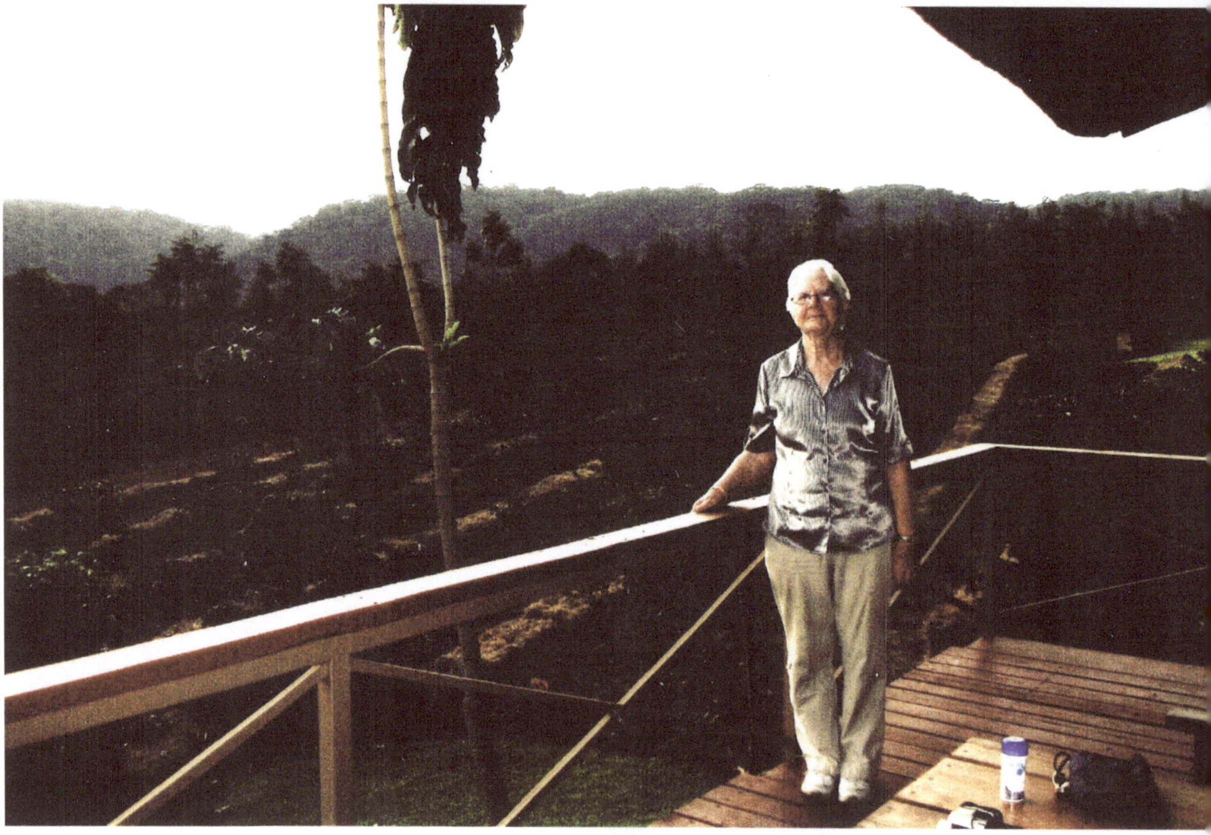

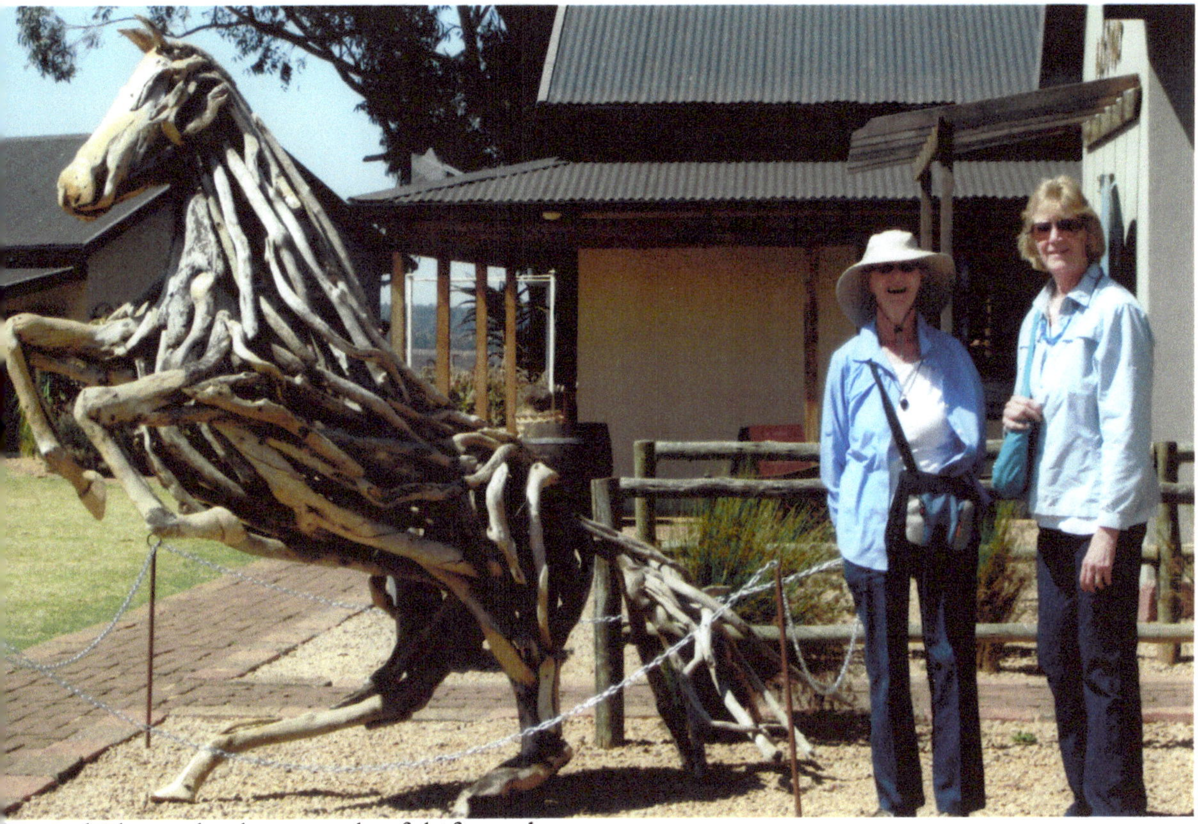

Una and Elin with a horse made of driftwood

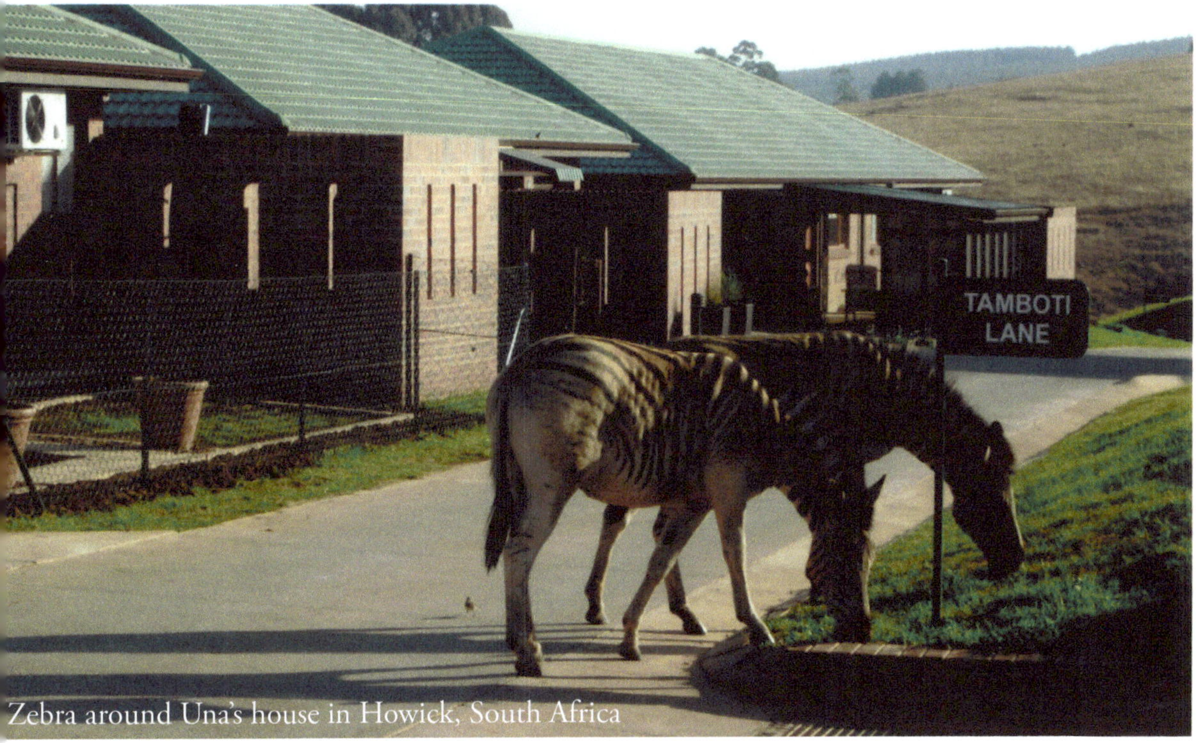

Zebra around Una's house in Howick, South Africa

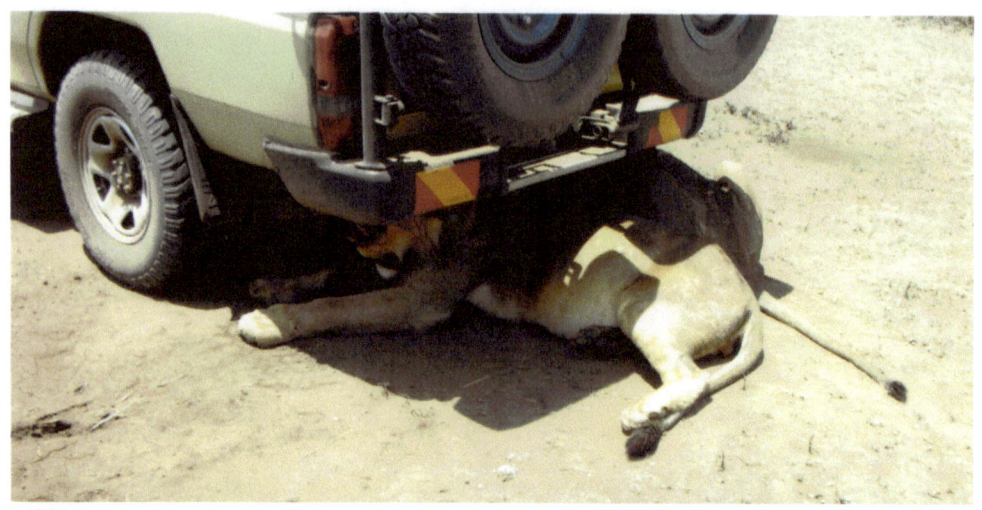

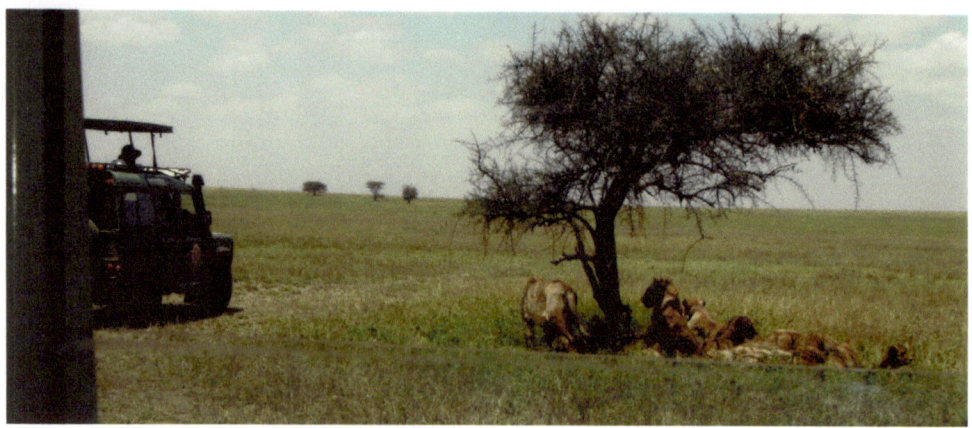

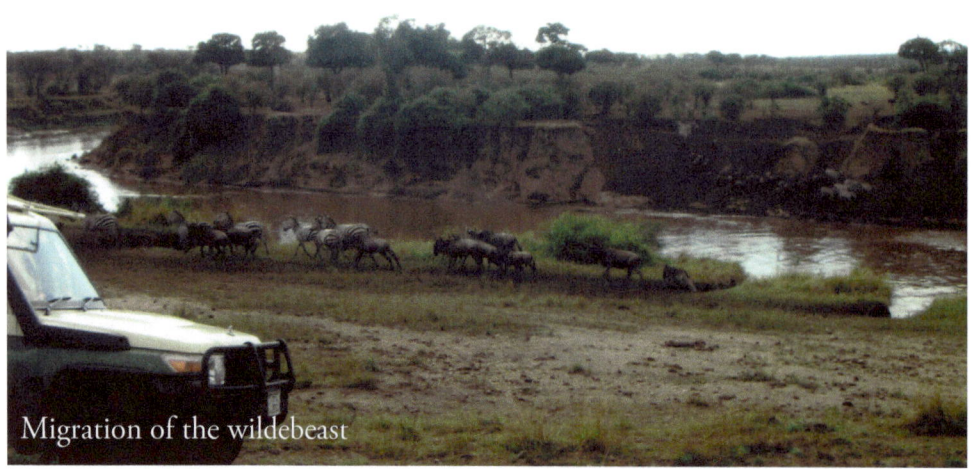
Migration of the wildebeast

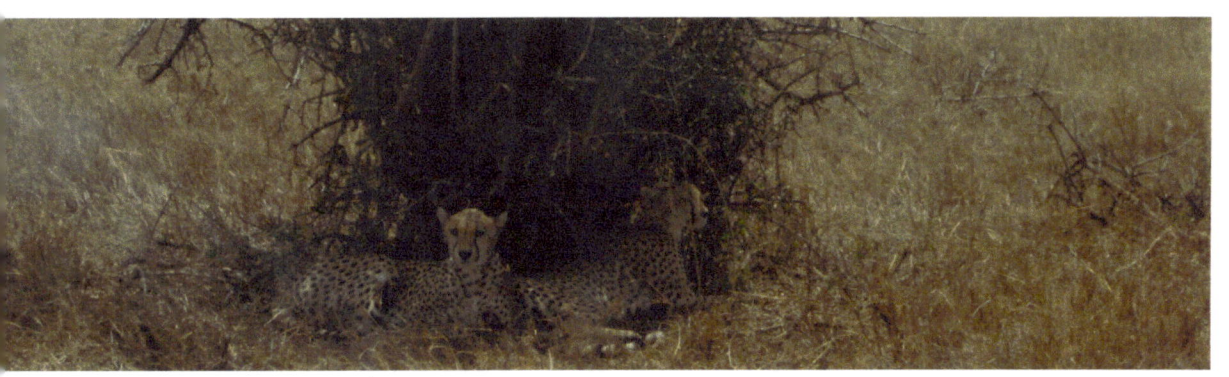
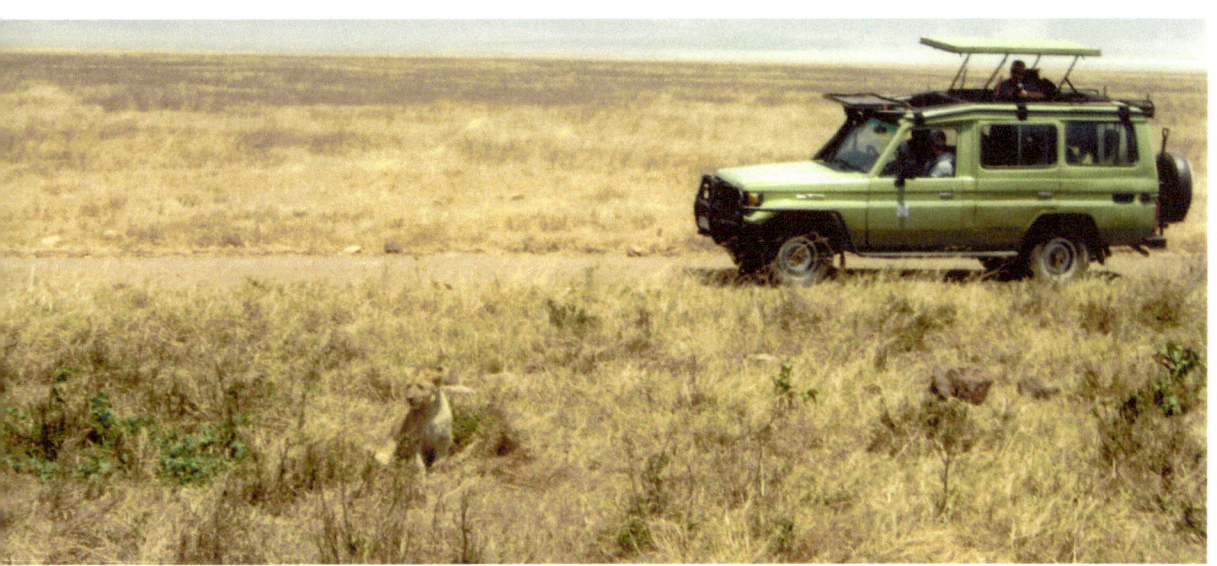
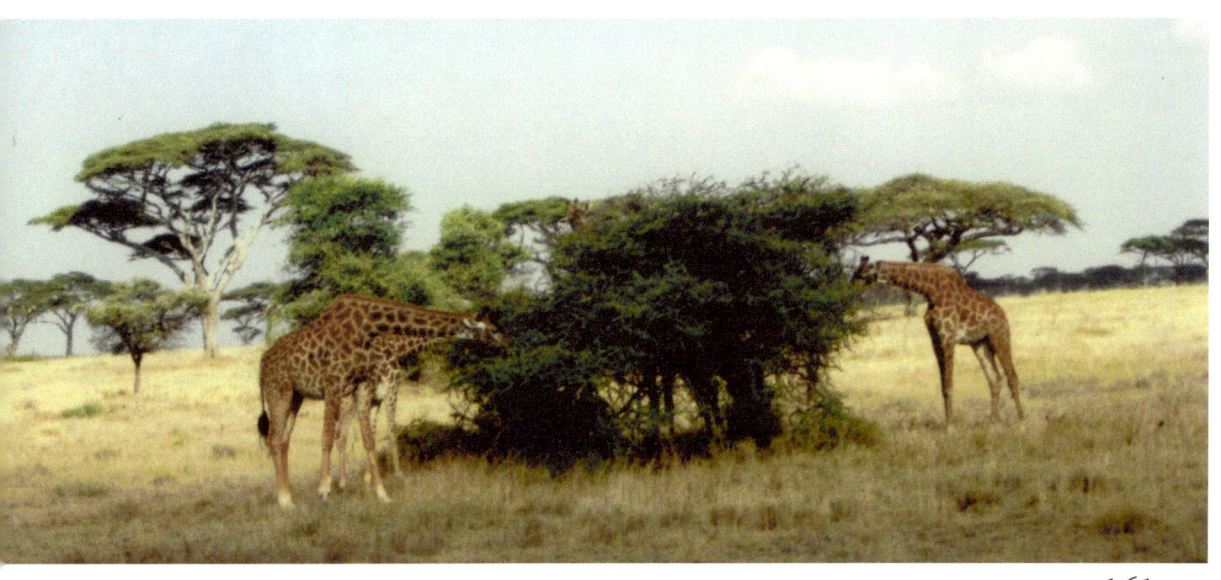

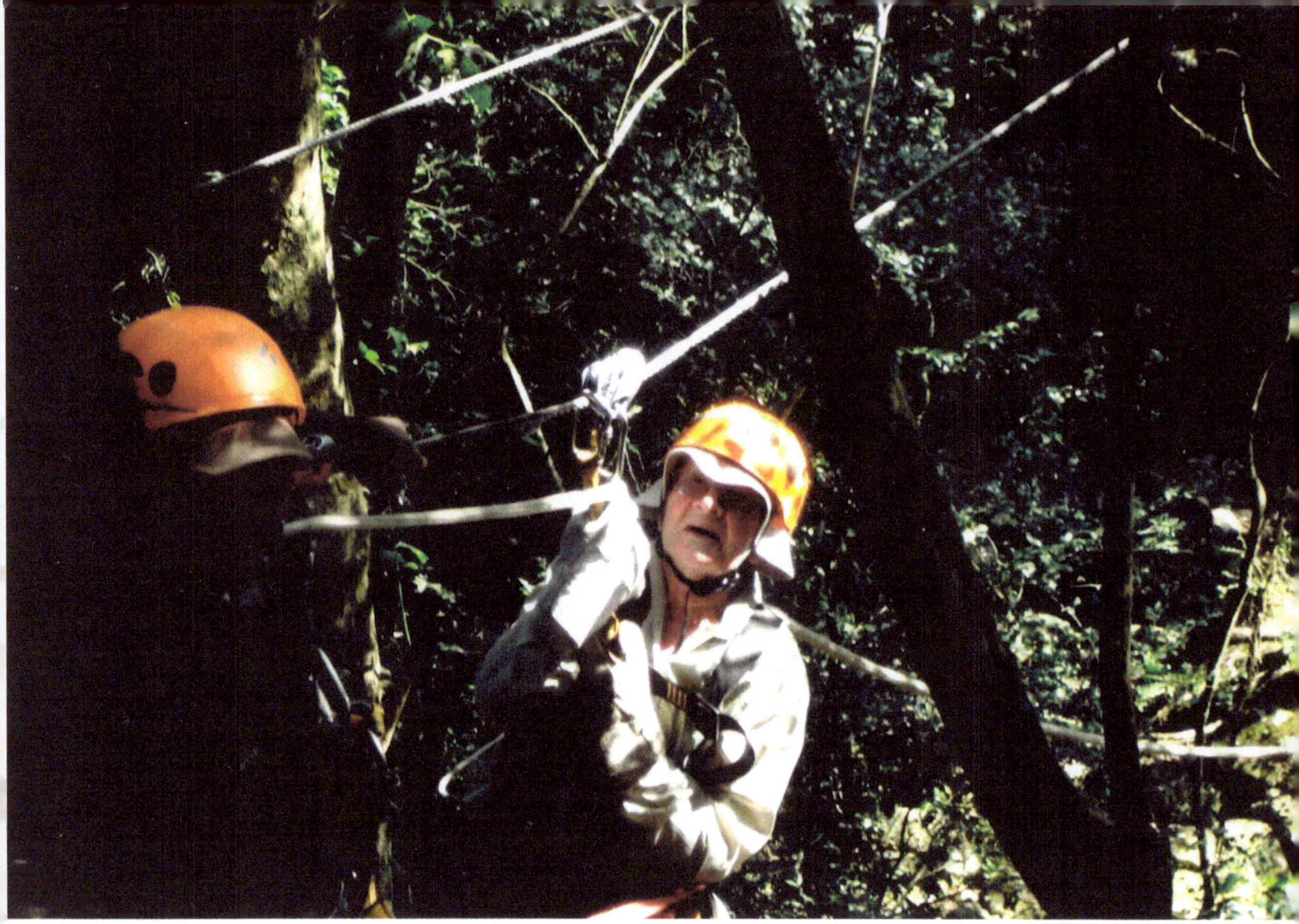

Ziplining near Howick, South Africa

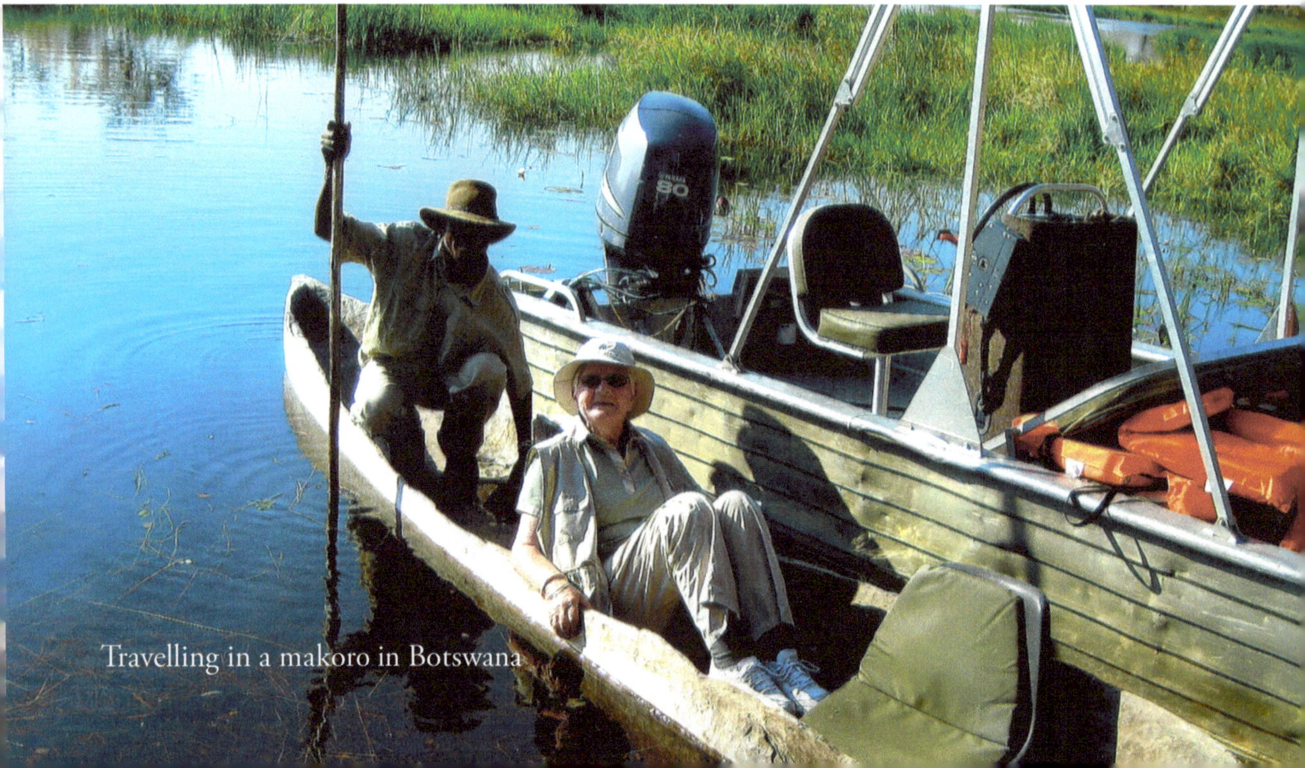

Travelling in a makoro in Botswana

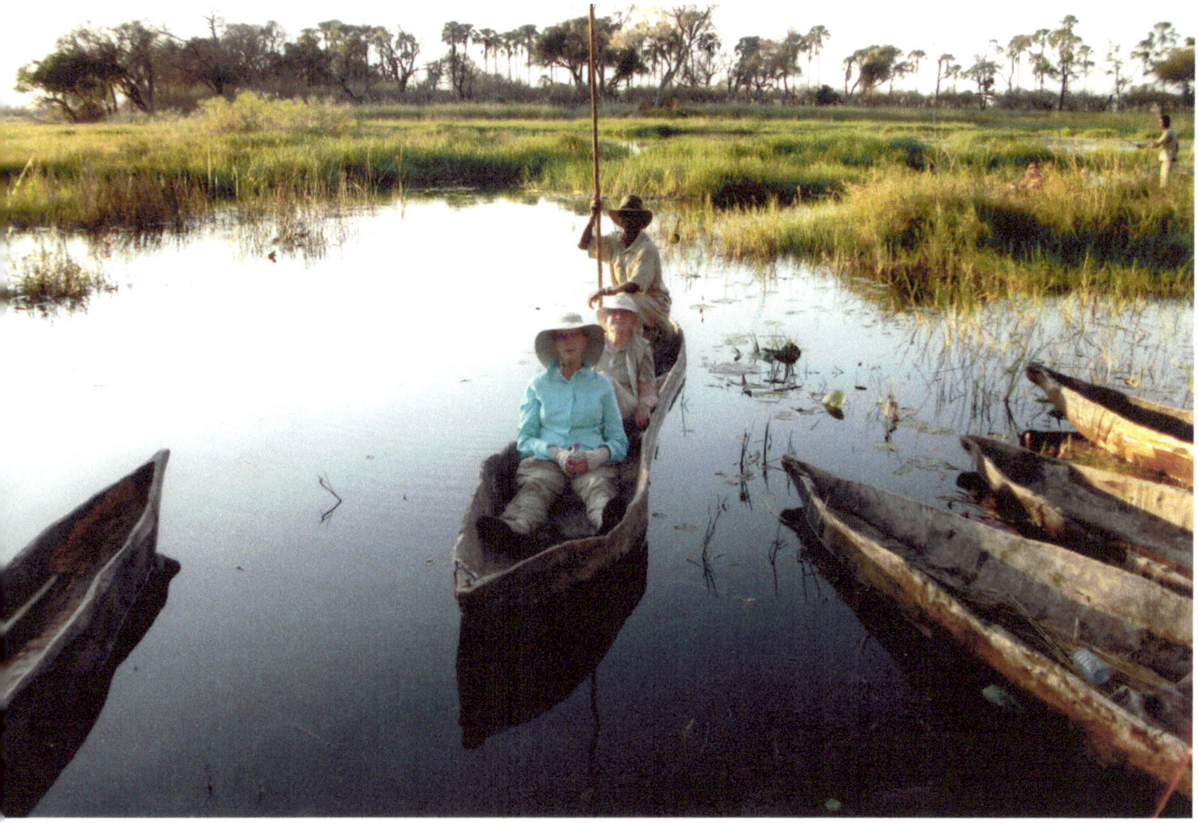

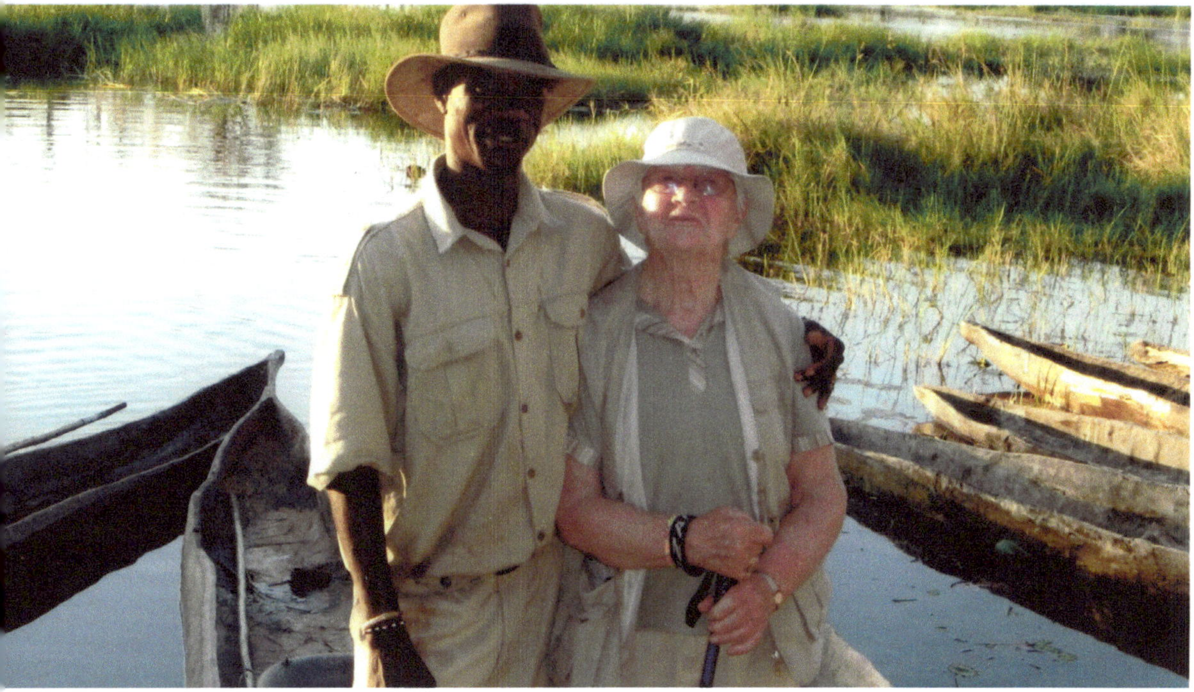

With our guide in Botswana

Victoria Falls

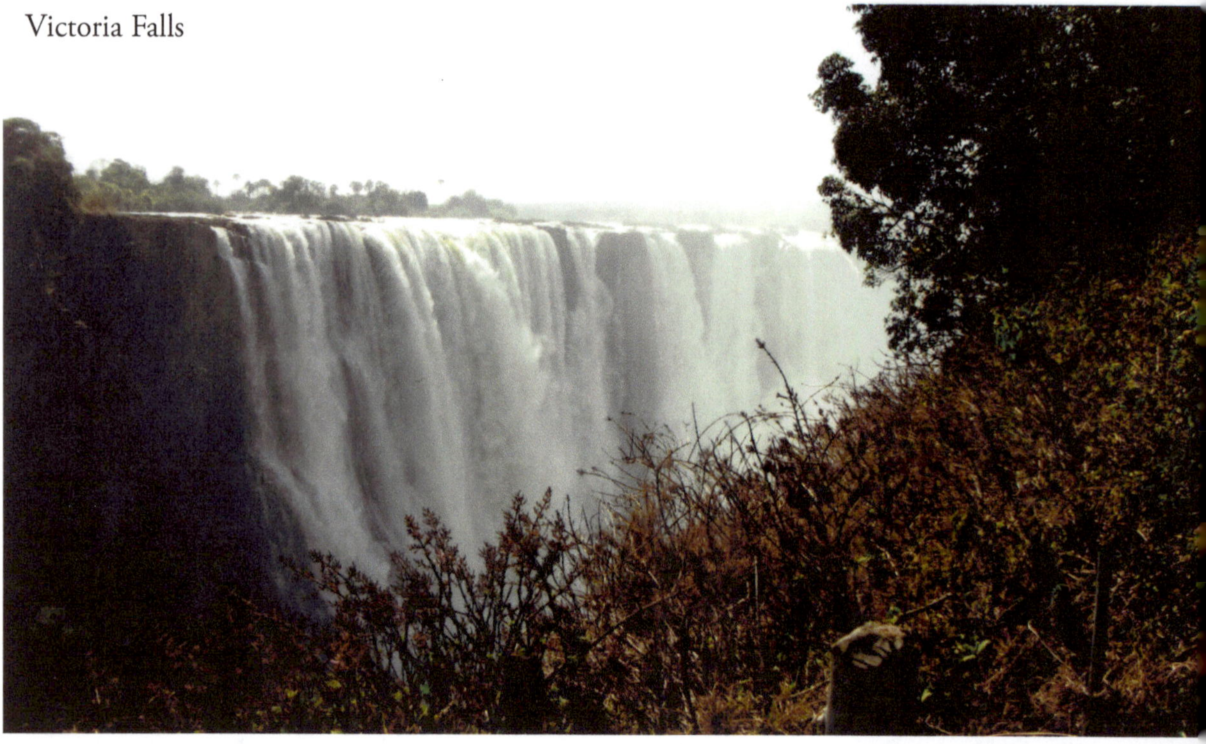

Me overlooking Victoria Falls

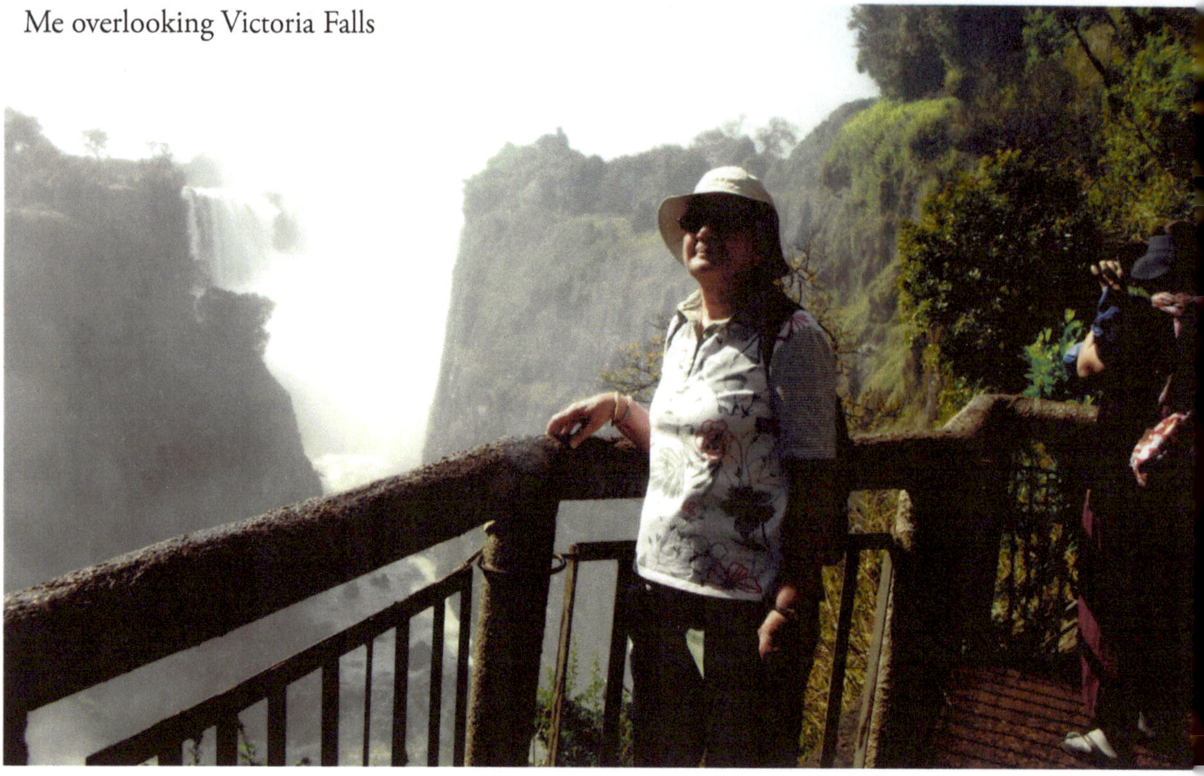

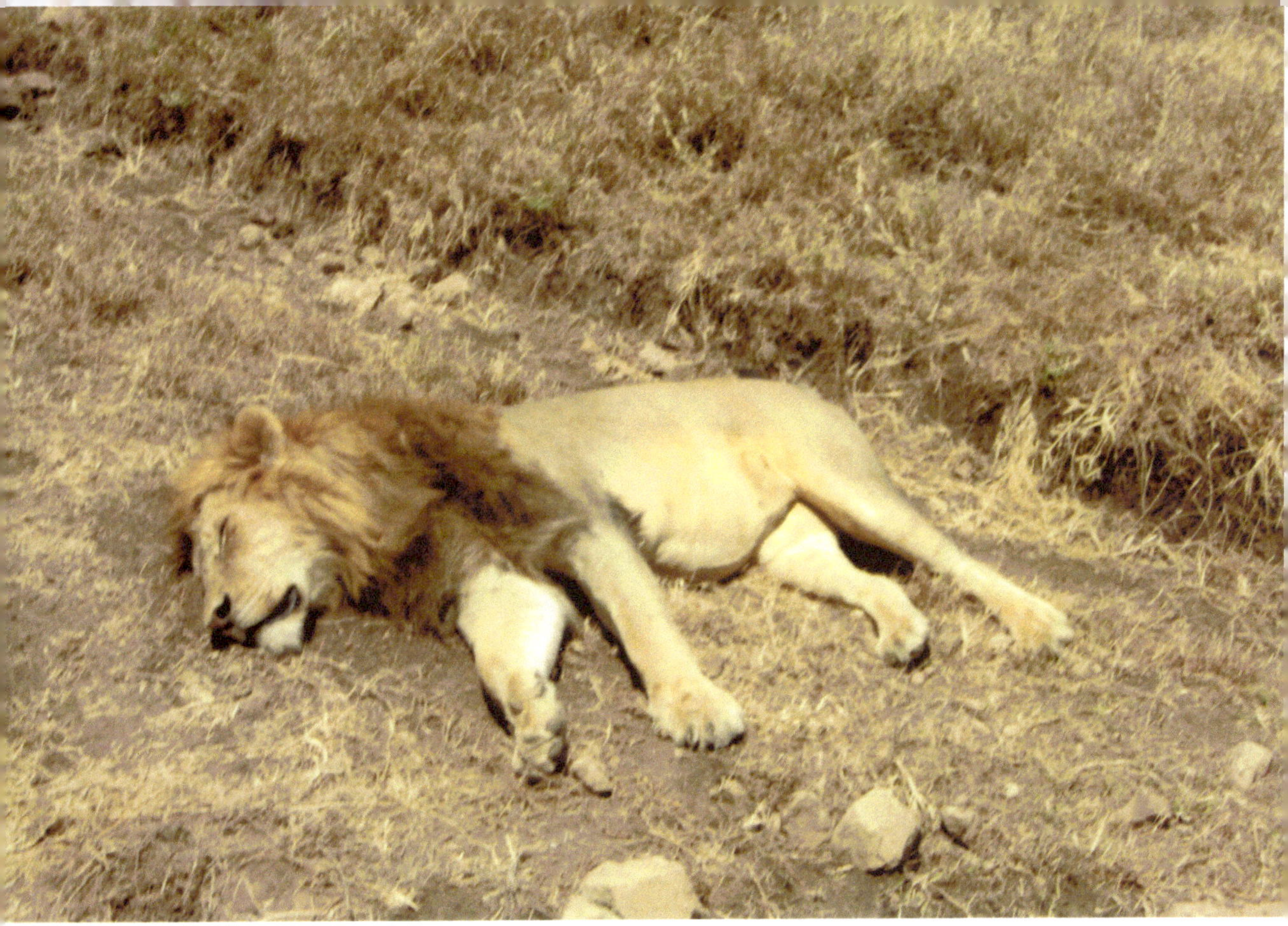

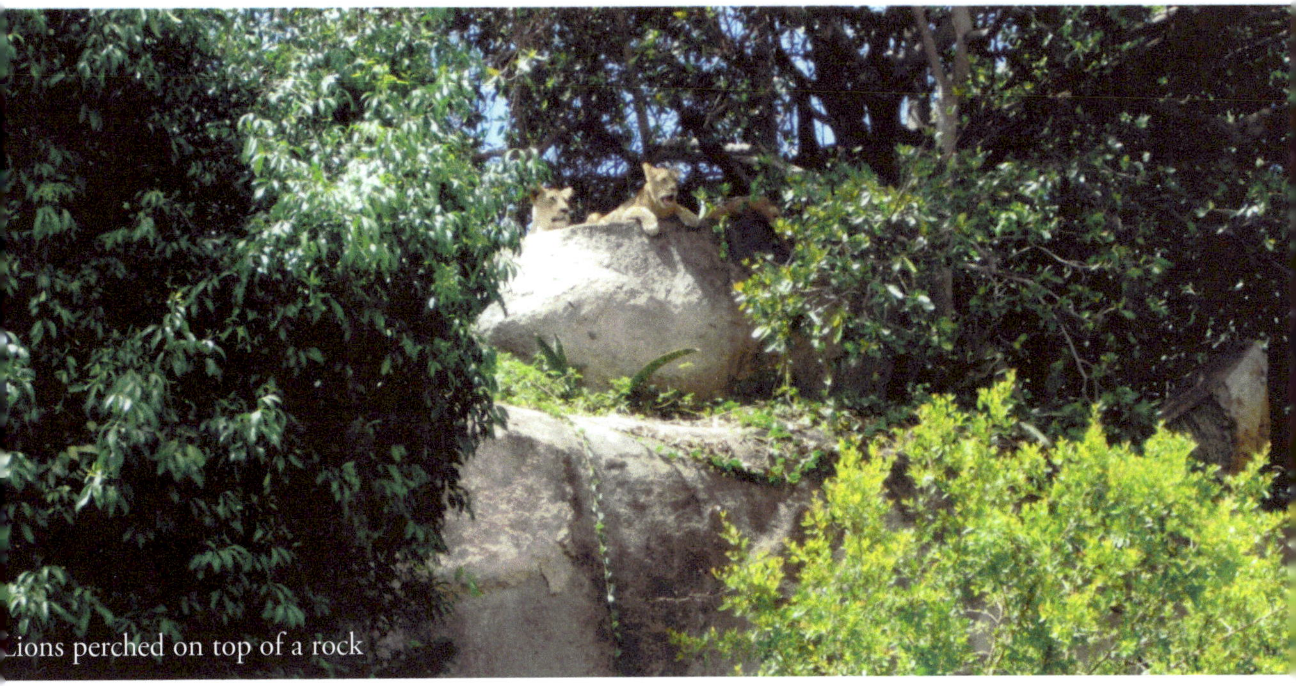

Lions perched on top of a rock

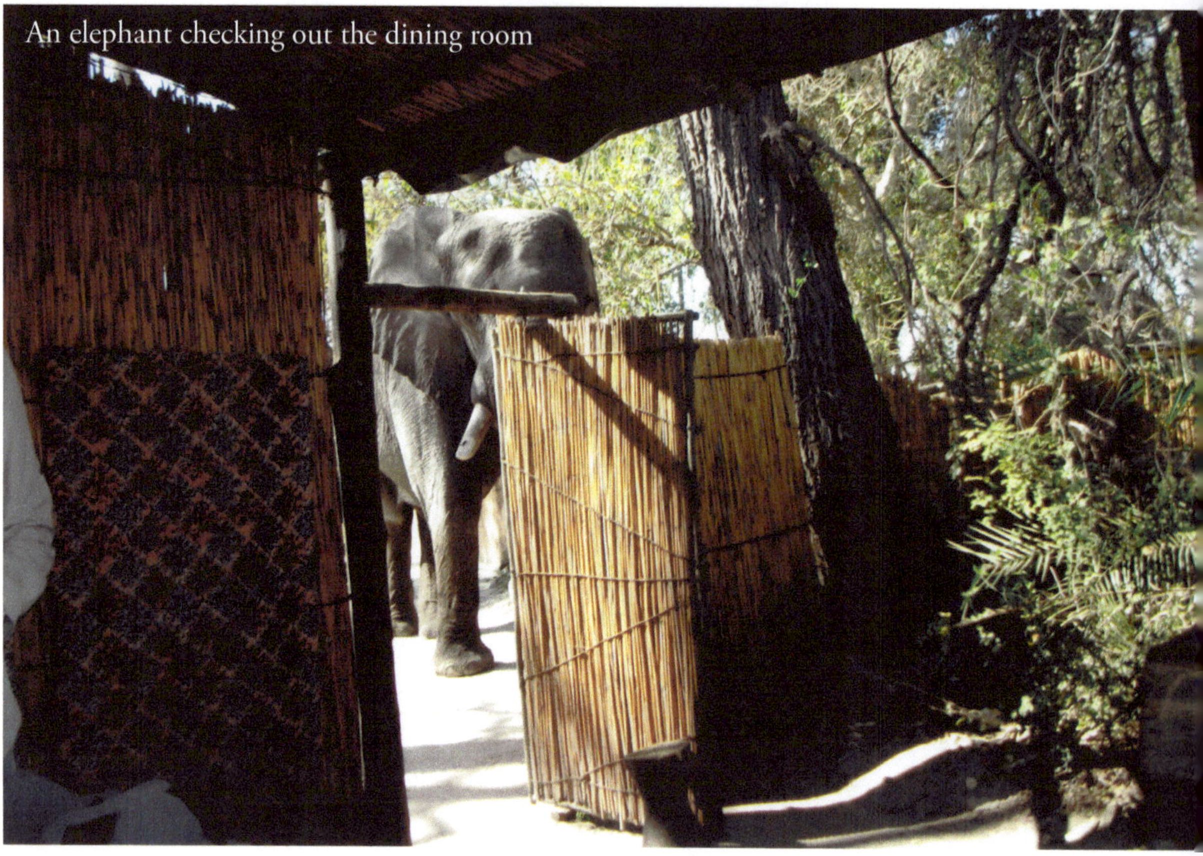

An elephant checking out the dining room

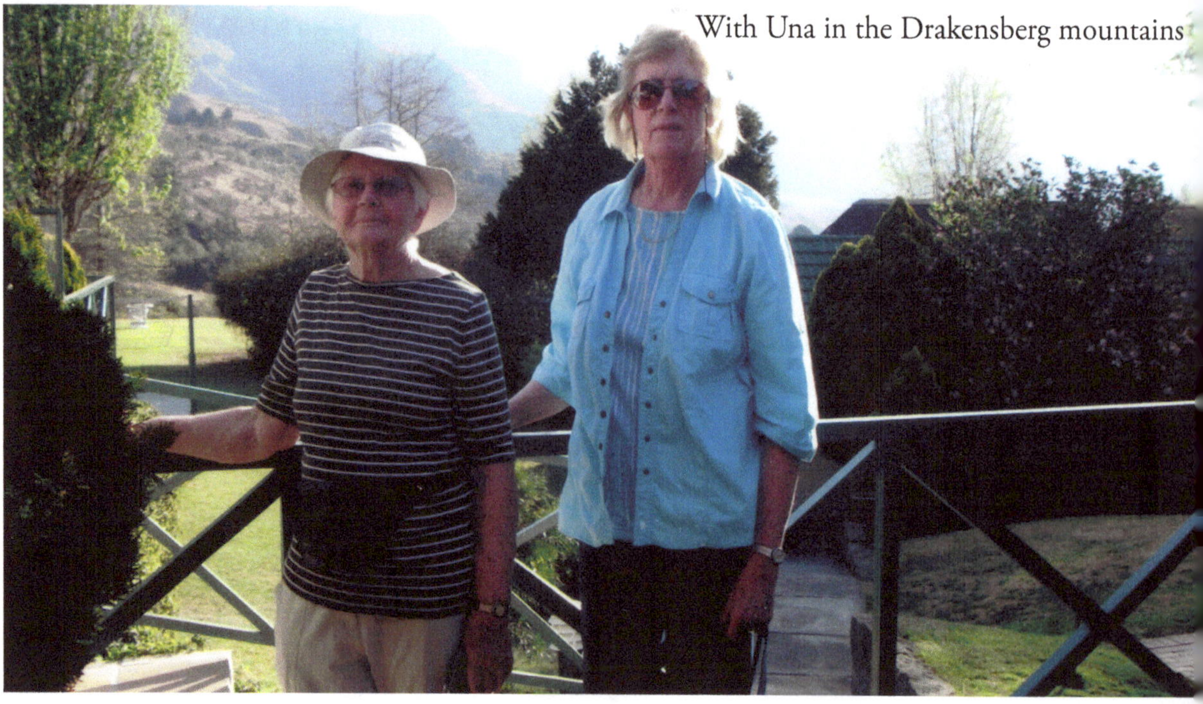

With Una in the Drakensberg mountains

It turned out much better than the Shongololo train safari could have been. The camps were great and not full. The guides were fantastic! The transport could not have been better. We travelled from one location to the next in small planes, where we were sometimes the only passengers. The same on the game drives. Typically six or more in a vehicle, yet we mostly had only one other couple, or we were the only ones. The driver would ask us what we wanted to see. Had we seen leopard yet? No? Then today we will see a leopard. We saw the big five, and the great migration of wildebeest and many birds as Elin has a great interest in birds, so the guide would always be on the lookout for unusual birds. It was the best of all the tours I have done.

It is always difficult to compare as each country has its charm and beauty, but we felt very glad that our train safari had been cancelled. This was just so special! We ended our holiday with a visit to Una in Howick where we spent time visiting the Drakensberg mountains. How very fortunate we were!

My next trip was to Ireland which I found interesting and after, as it is close to Holland I had to go and visit my family of course. Then in 2015 my friend Bi and I went to Alaska. I wanted to do the cruise of the inside passage but also wanted to see a bit more of the land. So, we booked a cruise and land tour with 'Princess'. The scenery both on the cruise and the land was amazing! Apart from the various optional tours in each harbour, we enjoyed the shows at night! Once you are elderly and don't drive at night anymore, you miss going to a good concert from time to time. That is why it is nifty that on the cruises there is a good show every night! No driving and included in the price. You can choose to go to the early show before dinner or to the later show after dinner.

I feel so blessed that I can enjoy my later years so much. This Alaska trip was spectacular. I could write pages on it as I have my diary with all the details. But if you are interested, go and do the cruise and land tour yourself. You won't be disappointed. The scenery is fantastic. The lodges are great in the national parks. We stayed in the Kenai National Park, The Denali National Park, The Wrangell St. Elias National Park which is the largest national park in North America. It is the size of Switzerland. The whole of Alaska has only 700,000 people with 1,500,000 visitors each summer.

We ended in Fairbanks from where we flew back to Vancouver. In

Tanzania, we saw a lot more game, but the scenery in Alaska beats even the scenery in China and Nepal. The staff in the lodges is mainly made up of students, mostly American, but also a few from Europe especially Eastern Europe. They pay for the program, which trains them for different kinds of jobs. Then while in Alaska they work for a small wage and board and lodging. They save their tips, and after four months they travel for a month (the Europeans I spoke to do this). Some Americans (non-students) go from here to the ski resorts where they take up work.

TRAVEL IN GENERAL

I have learned a thing or two about travel during my life. If you like adventure travel, you should look at companies that specialise in this. Consider your age as some companies won't take you over a certain age. Naturally, you are dependent on your budget. Some outstanding companies are not expensive as long as you don't mind roughing it a bit. World Expedition is good, and so is Peregrine.

I travelled to India in 2007 with my sister in law, who lives in Washington D.C. with Imaginative Travel and found them very good too. We saw a lot of Rajasthan and also of the North such as Shimla and Manali from where you have beautiful views of the Himalayas.

These were usually package deals, so you could not choose your airline, and therefore I have never benefited from frequent flyer points, although I am a member of Qantas and Malaysian Airways. So, I have never had a free flight. Once I was upgraded to business class on a flight from Amsterdam to Singapore, which was delightful.

But, would I ever pay for a business class flight? No way! The difference in price is so not worth it. Once you get old like I am now, you can book 'assisted passenger', and you don't have to queue at the customs or at the carousel to wait for your luggage. I have done it twice now and won't travel any other way.

For a long flight such as to Europe consider an overnight stop. I did that last year on my trip to Amsterdam. I flew with Etihad to Abu Dhabi and spent two nights there. I was able to see the mosque and the new Louvre, and also take a hop on hop off bus tour and did a desert safari. All in all, a lovely break and then flew to Amsterdam arriving fresh and well. No jetlag! And a lot cheaper than business class! I even had three seats to myself for the longest flight from Perth to Abu Dhabi which is eleven hours, and could lie down. The plane was not very full, and many people had extra seats. The flight from Abu Dhabi to Amsterdam was full, but that was only seven hours.

When you choose your seat, consider if you need to use the bathroom a lot. If you do, choose an aisle seat, so you do not have to disturb your neighbours. If not, pick a window seat as you have a little more space to sleep as you can put your pillow against the window.

I always pack soft things (clothes) in my hand luggage and put this under my feet as my feet tend to swell up a lot during a long flight.

Some people say you should not recline your seat as it is not fair to the person behind you. I don't agree. As long as you straighten up at mealtimes. If the person in front of you does not straighten up at mealtimes, don't sulk, just tap them on the shoulder and ask politely if they would, and most of the time you find that they just forgot. The cabin crew should ask them, but they don't always.

REFLECTIONS ON MY LIFE SO FAR

Sometimes people ask me if I am rich. Money wise no, I am an aged pensioner, although I am lucky to get a small pension from Holland and a minimal pension from France. But yes, I feel very rich to be in good health and able to follow my dreams. I will travel for as long my old body lets me. I have a loving family here in Australia with three children and their partners, twelve grandchildren and two great-grandchildren, not bad considering I had my first child at the age of thirty-five. So yes, I am very well-off! Not forgetting my family in Canada and in Holland and my in-laws in South Africa, where I always feel so warmly welcome whenever I visit.

In 2016 I went with my friend Bi to Spain, Portugal and Morocco. After which Bi wanted to visit her sister in Denmark, but did not want to travel back to Australia by herself. Her sister and husband very kindly invited me to come with Bi which I accepted gracefully. However, my time in Denmark did not turn out so good, as I got the shingles. Fortunately, I was diagnosed within the seventy-two hours of the start of the rash, so I could get the medication and was feeling much better within two weeks. I had been feeling fatigued during

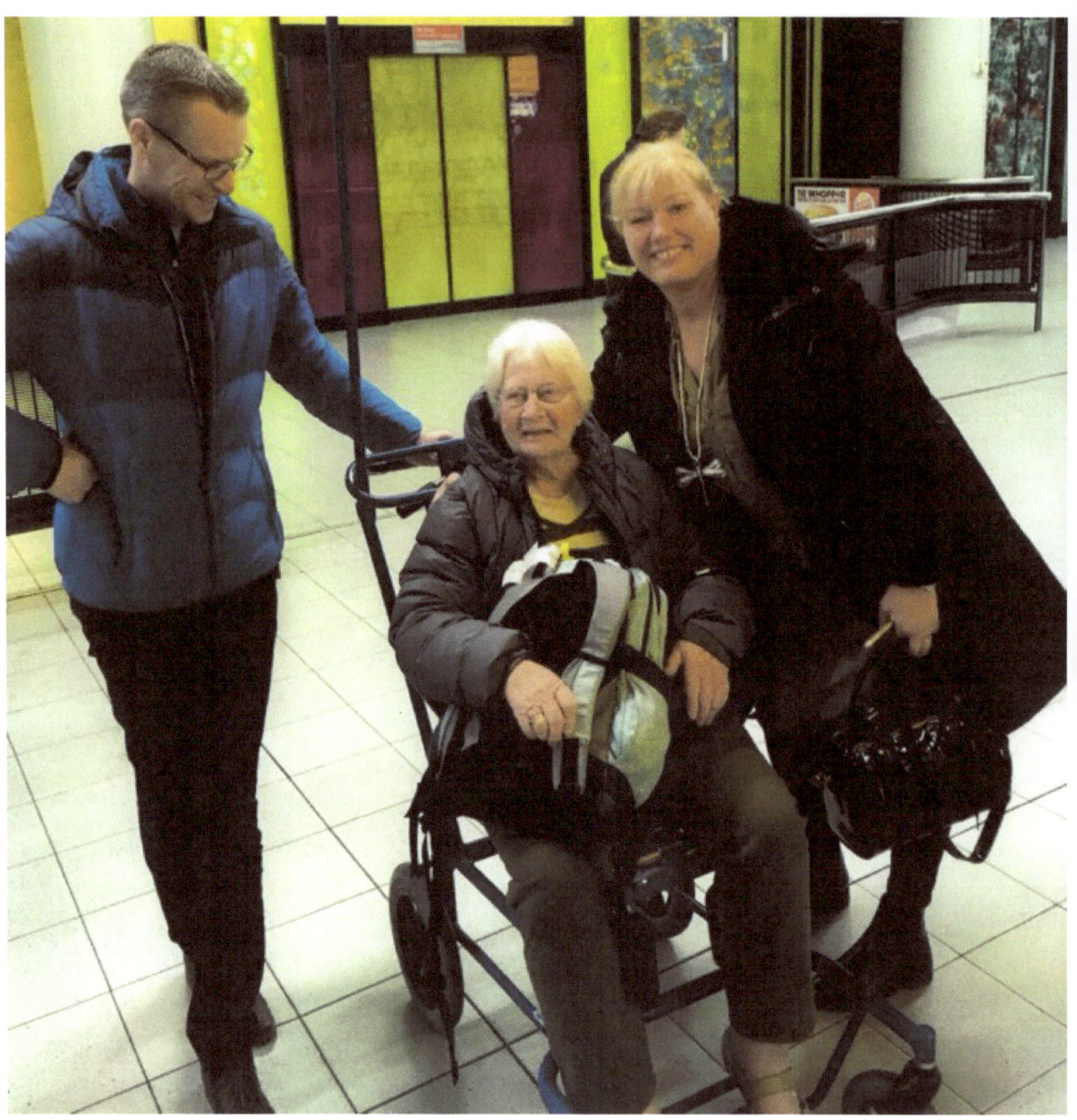

Me at the airport, the chair is included in assisted passage

that holiday and often stayed on the coach because I did not feel up to the sightseeing. In hindsight, I might already have had an underworking thyroid gland, which was diagnosed later. Since being on medication, I feel normal again.

The cruise I took around Japan in 2017 was very enjoyable. We cruised with Princess again, and both Bi and I found Japan very interesting and safe.

When in a big city like Tokyo or Osaka you see this mass of pedestrians as most people use public transport to get to work. With that many trains amd buses, there is no need for a car, so the traffic is not bad in spite of the millions of people living in the big cities. Most men seem to wear white shirts with black pants, so it looks like everyone is in uniform. All wear shoes, no sandals or thongs here. You pick out the visitors by their dress. Very formal. They don't accept tips, and if a taxi driver quotes you a price and at the end of the journey the meter shows less than the quote, he only takes the meter price. They are a very polite and helpful people and very honest too. If you leave your purse by mistake after having a coffee it will still be there when you come back an hour later. We loved Japan as we felt so safe as two elderly ladies at night out on the streets.

In October 2017 my niece Loes, (the daughter of my eldest brother) rang me as her mum and dad were both turning ninety, to ask if I would come over? I had not planned to go again as the long journey is getting very tiring, I thought about it and decided ninety is very special, I should go. She suggested that I don't tell them or anyone else that I was coming as she wanted it to be a surprise. The party was going to be two weeks after their birthdays, so I sent them both cards and phoned each of them on their birthday, so they would not suspect anything. Well, you should have seen their faces when they saw me. They could not believe it and were so happy, that I was glad I had made the journey. I had booked 'assisted passage' so I did not have to wait so long at customs or the carousel for my luggage. I had also scheduled a stopover in Abu Dhabi so the journey was fine. I spent a lovely two weeks with the family who went out of their way to make my stay special. Frans and his wife Truus are both still in great shape. Living independently and managing shopping, cooking and general living very well. They still go to the gym once a week!

I have now come to the end of my book.

It is now 2018, and I have already booked a cruise around New Zealand with Bi in March as she has not been there. I have done a land tour of both islands with Brian, but a cruise will be different. I have last week gone back to play golf which I had stopped when the Armadale course closed because of redevelopment. The club kept playing at Marri Park (further away), and I found the drive there uncomfortable, so I stopped playing. However, the new course at Armadale is now finished, so as long the weather is not too hot I intend to play again.

I have also booked a train trip on the Indian Pacific to Sydney in May. I have saved these trips including the Ghan to Darwin and the Indian Pacific till I was old. I think I qualify now! I have turned eighty-four in December. I have at present three of my grandchildren living with me. Four years ago, Jessie, one of Wendy's girls, asked if she could stay with me. She had been working in Brookton at the nursing home in the kitchen but wanted a change. She could get a job at McDonald's. She has since worked herself up to a managerial position.

Then nearly three years ago Max, one of Wendy's boys asked if he could stay, as he was working as an apprentice panel beater in Perth and had been getting to and from Perth to Brookton with his dad previously, but now his dad had found work closer to home. He will be finishing his apprenticeship in May and will come with me on the Indian Pacific tour to Sydney.

Then last year Kody, his brother asked if he could stay. As I have only a small three-bedroom unit, I said, "you are most welcome, but I have not got a room for you. For the time being, You will have to sleep on the couch, until we sort something out." Max suggested a bunk bed, but I hate bunk beds as they are so hard to make up, so I said, "lets measure if we can fit another bed in your room." That worked, and Bi helped out by lending me a perfect field bed. So, although it is a bit of a squeeze, they all have a place to stay. The boys go home on the weekend. Jessie does not get many weekends off and often remains in Perth on her days off. She enjoys some social life and likes going out with her friends.

When people ask me, "is it not too much for you?" I say, "not really, as they are at work all day and although I do their washing and cook for them, they keep me company, and it keeps me young." I enjoy having them and get a break on weekends, so life is good and I am happy to be able to help out. They help me with some things that are getting hard for me such as some pruning and weeding in the garden. As I am no friend of my computer, it is nice to have their help. They can and will cook whenever I ask them, but as they come home at around 6 pm. I like to have dinner soon after, so I cook most of the time.

As I look back on my life and all the amazing adventures I have had, I feel I have lived a most interesting life and am grateful that I have reached such a wonderful old age with good health, a beautiful family and dear friends.

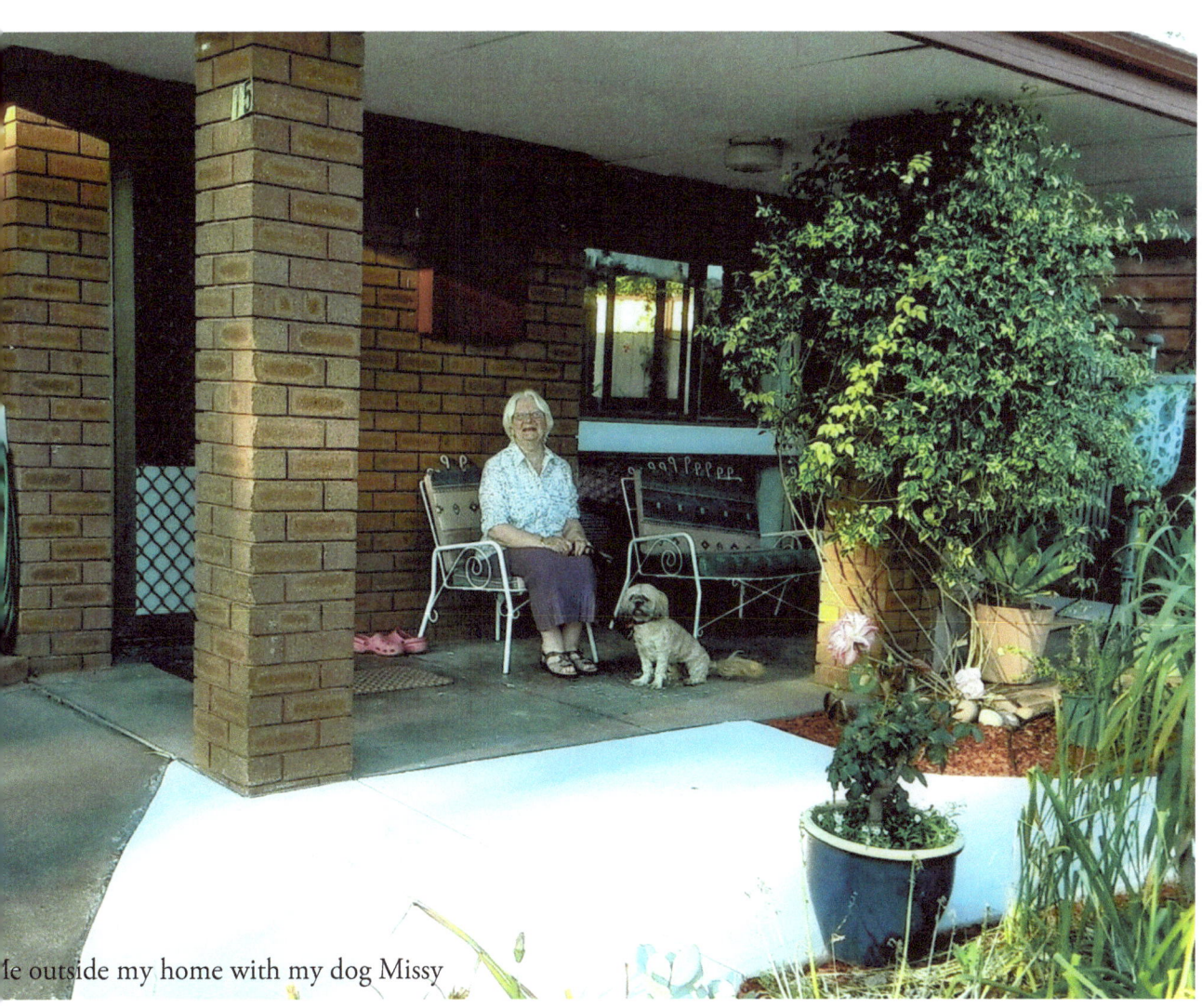

Me outside my home with my dog Missy

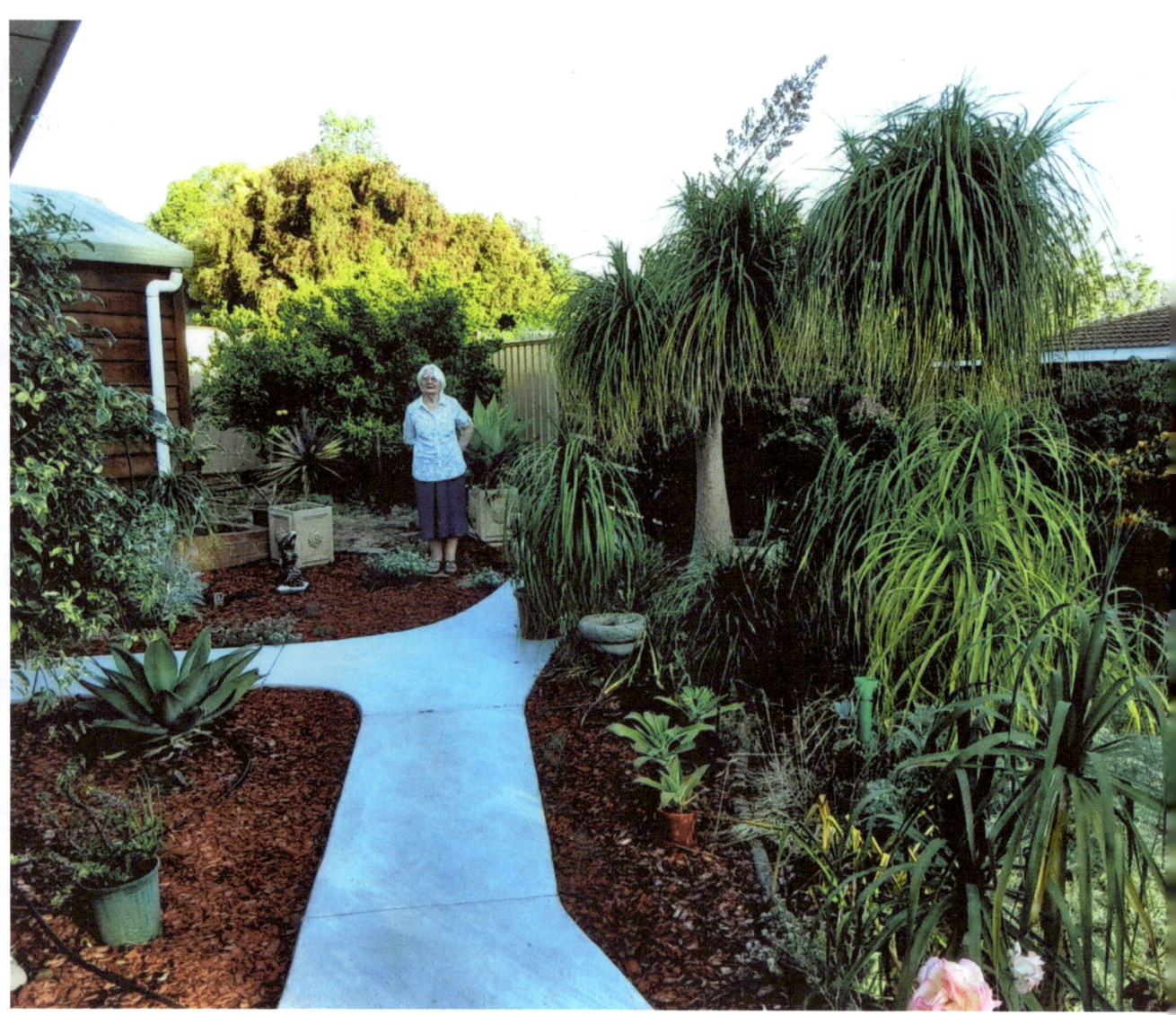
Me in my garden

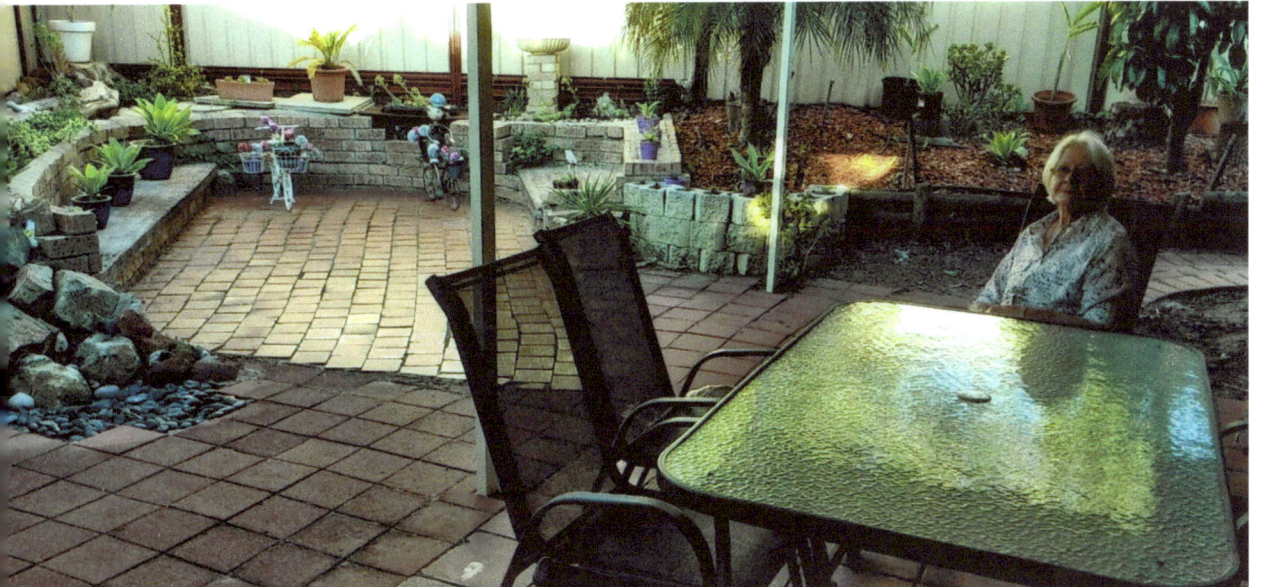

My backyard

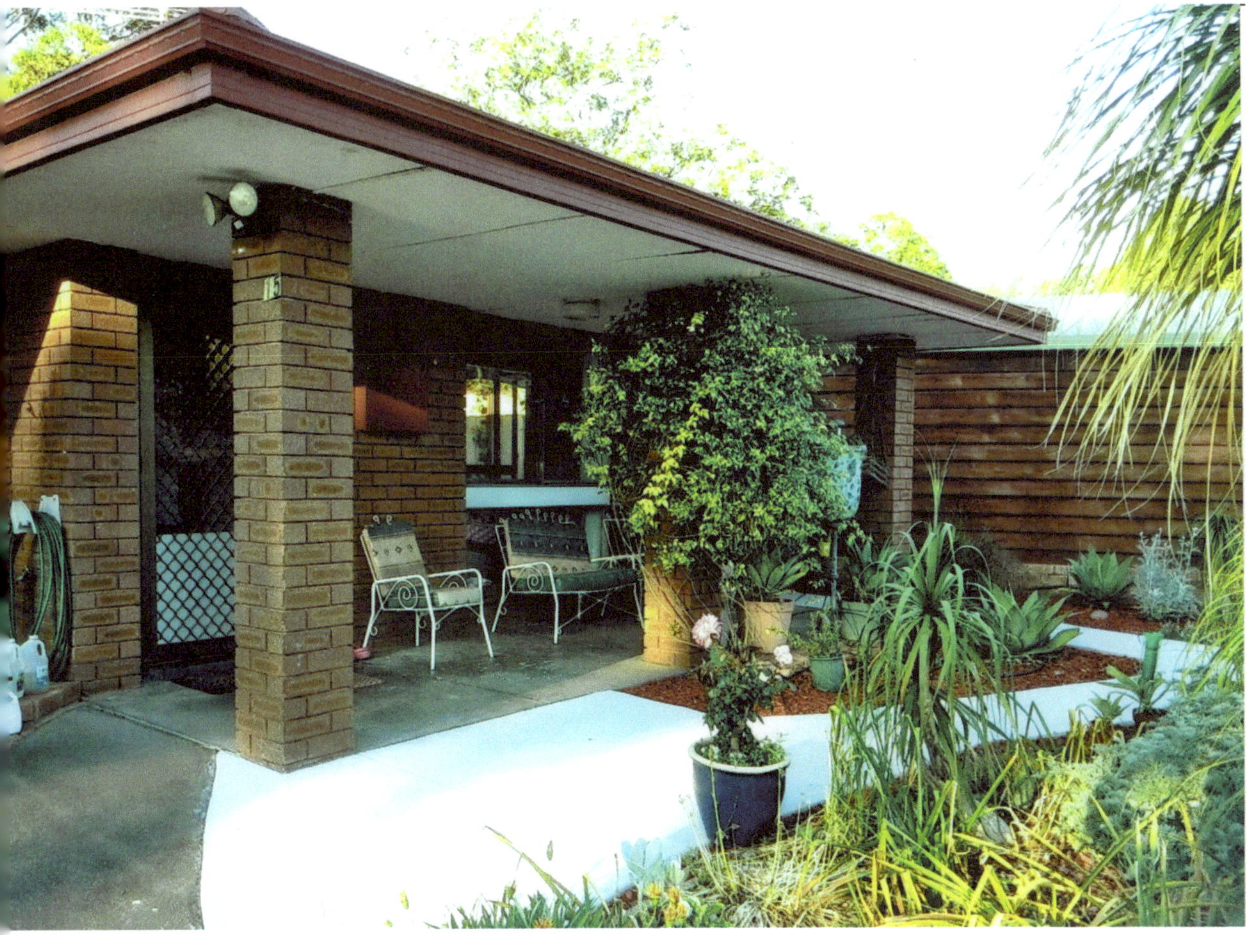

My home

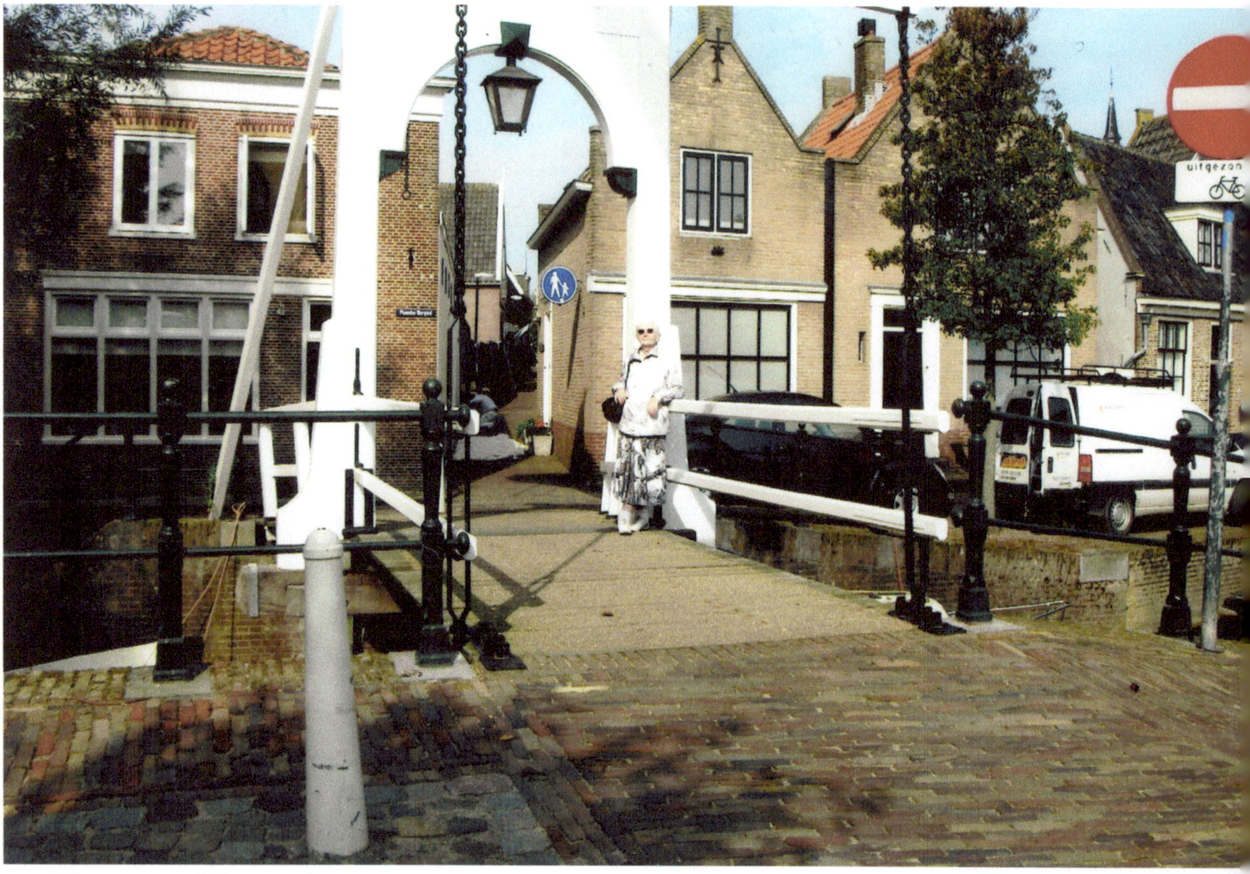

Me in central Amsterdam

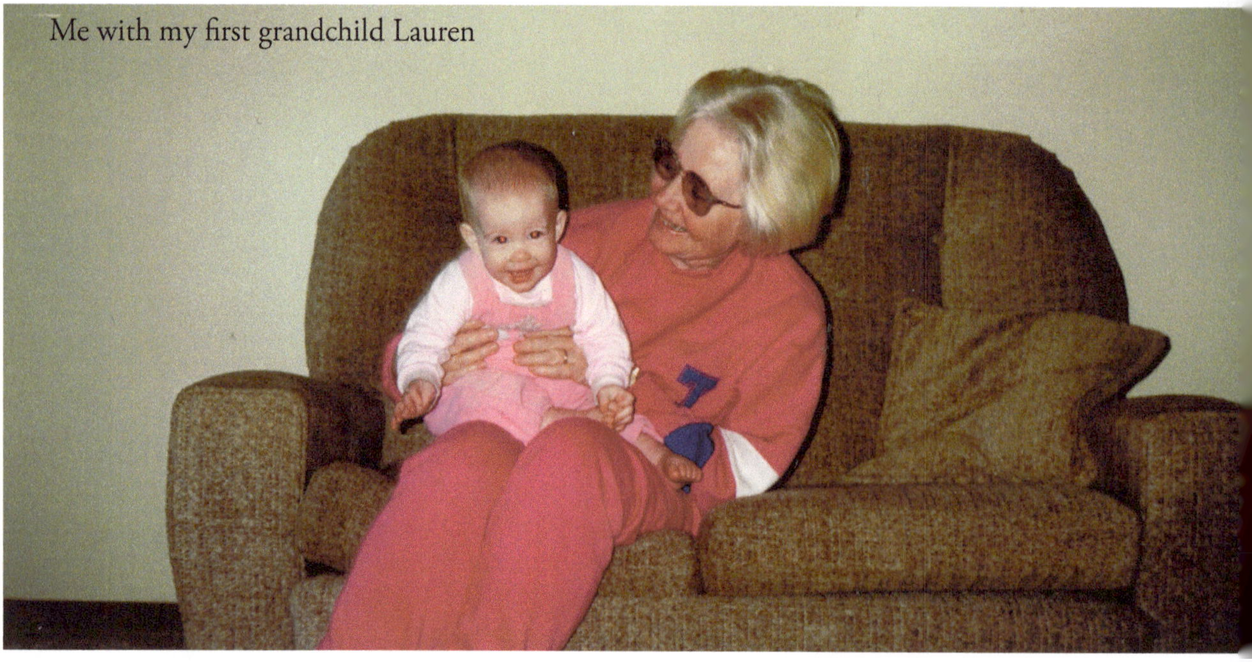

Me with my first grandchild Lauren

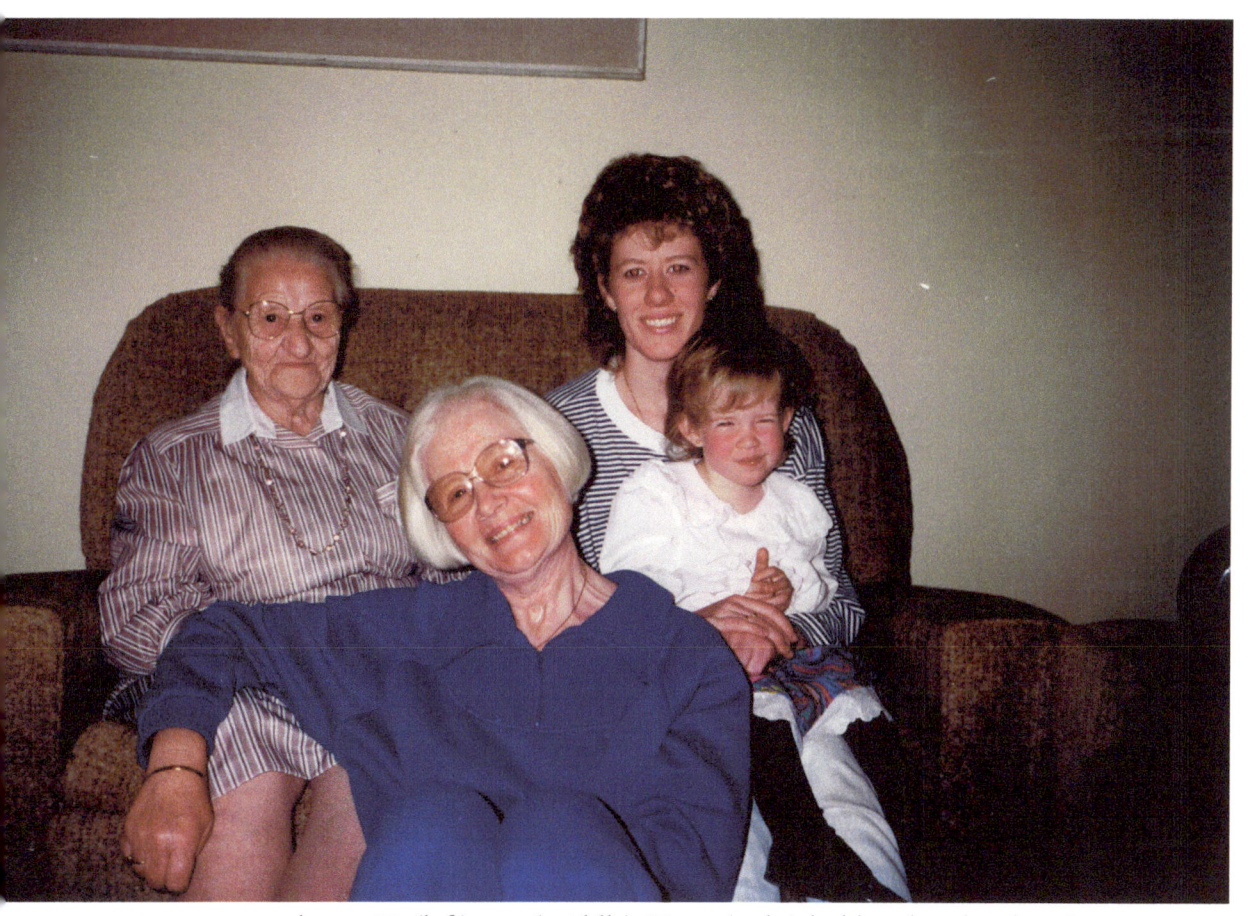
Four generations, my mother at 90 (left), me (middle), Tracy (right) holding her daughter Lauren

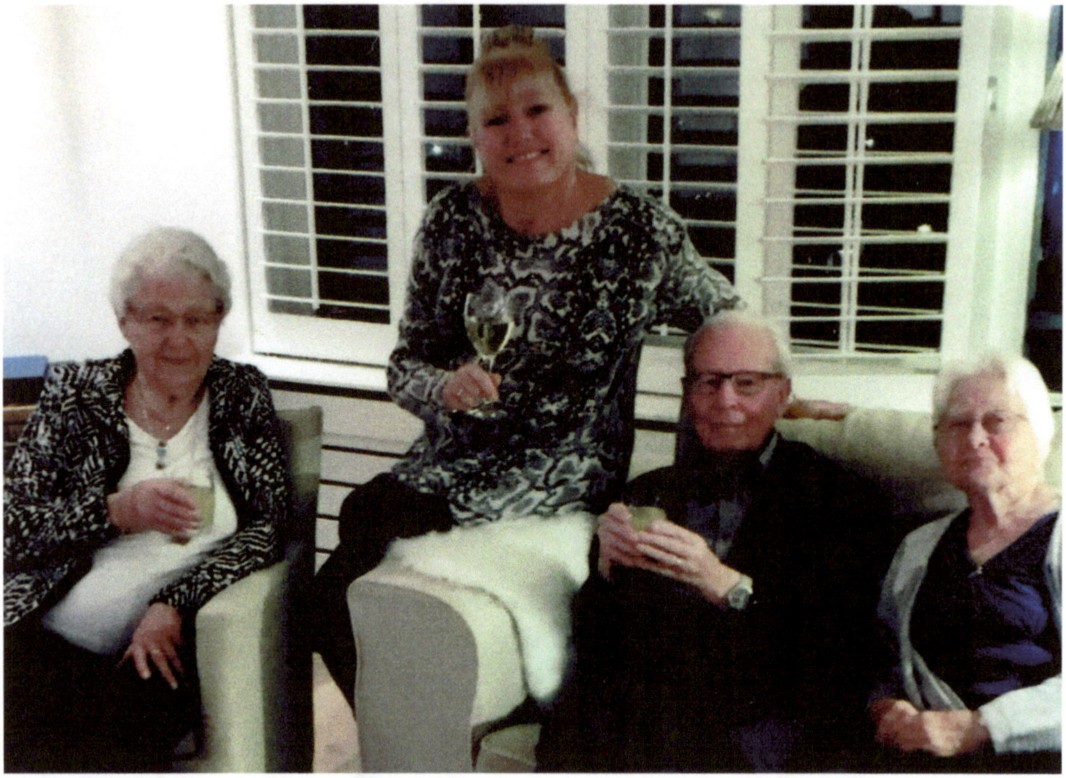

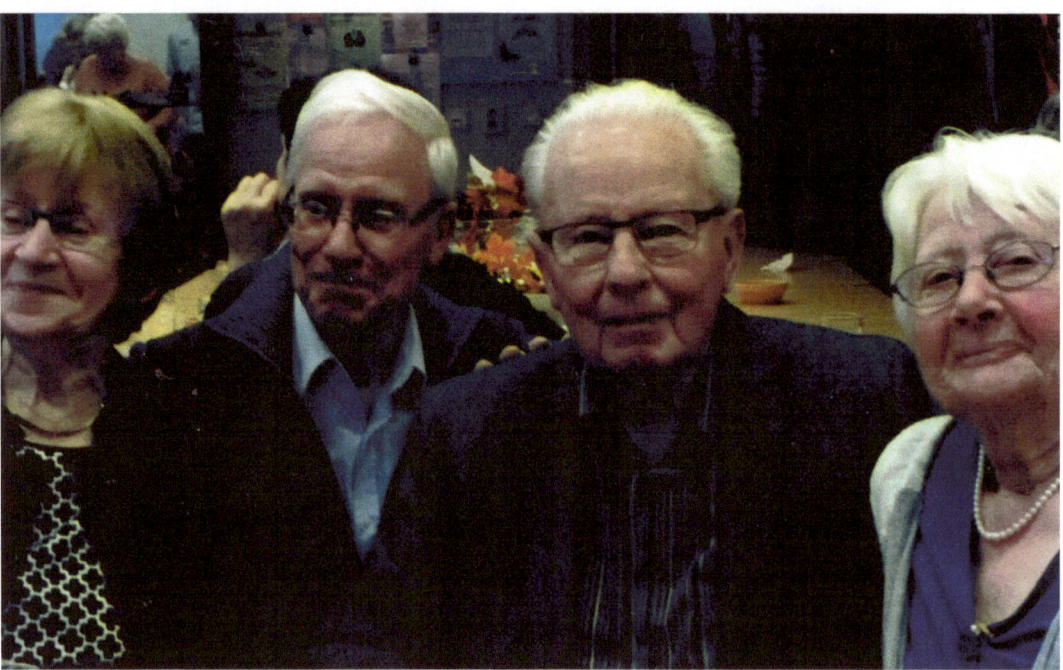

Truus (left), Loes, Frans and me (right)

Ans (left), Faas, Frans and me (right); four of the five siblings still alive in 2018

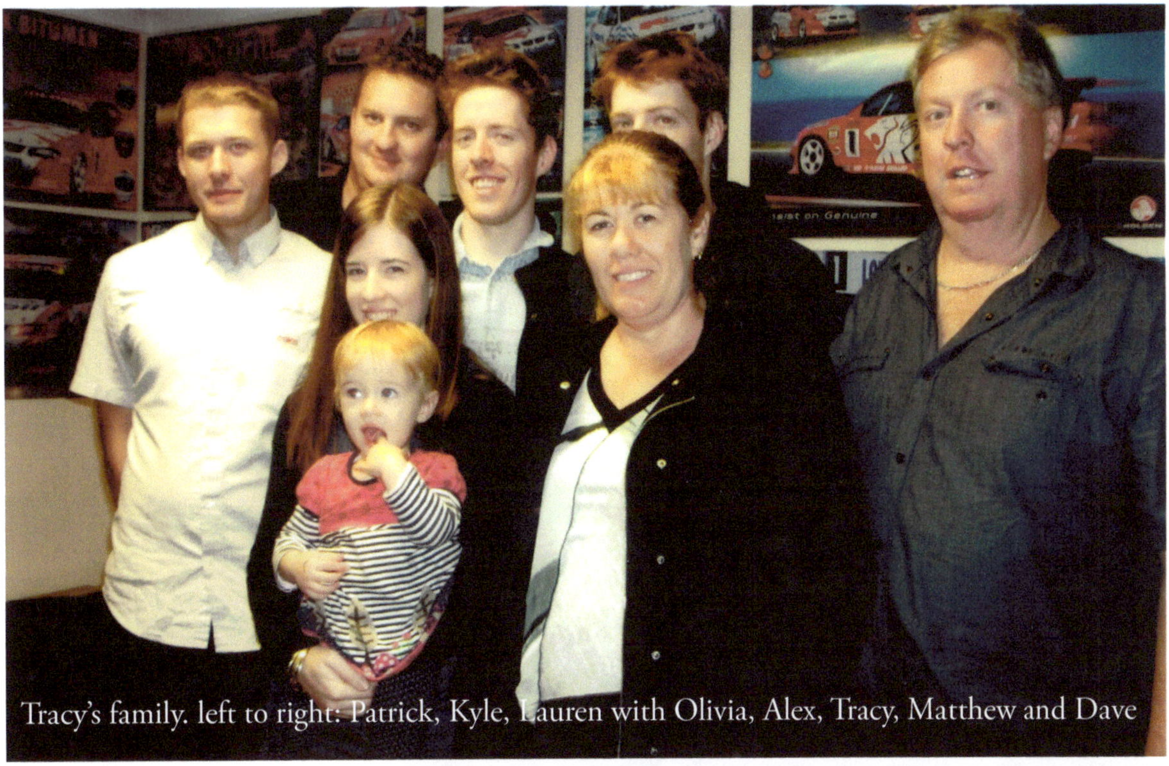

Tracy's family. left to right: Patrick, Kyle, Lauren with Olivia, Alex, Tracy, Matthew and Dave

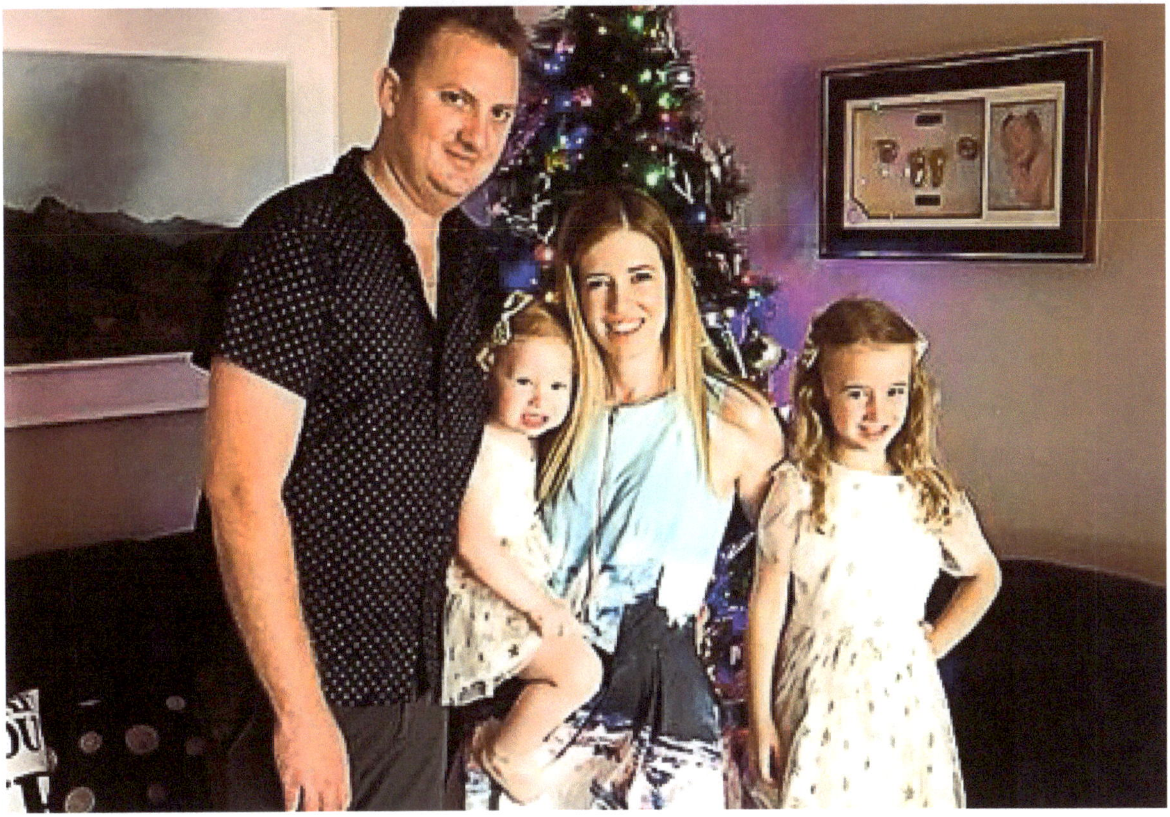

Left to right: Kyle, Eva, Lauren and Olivia

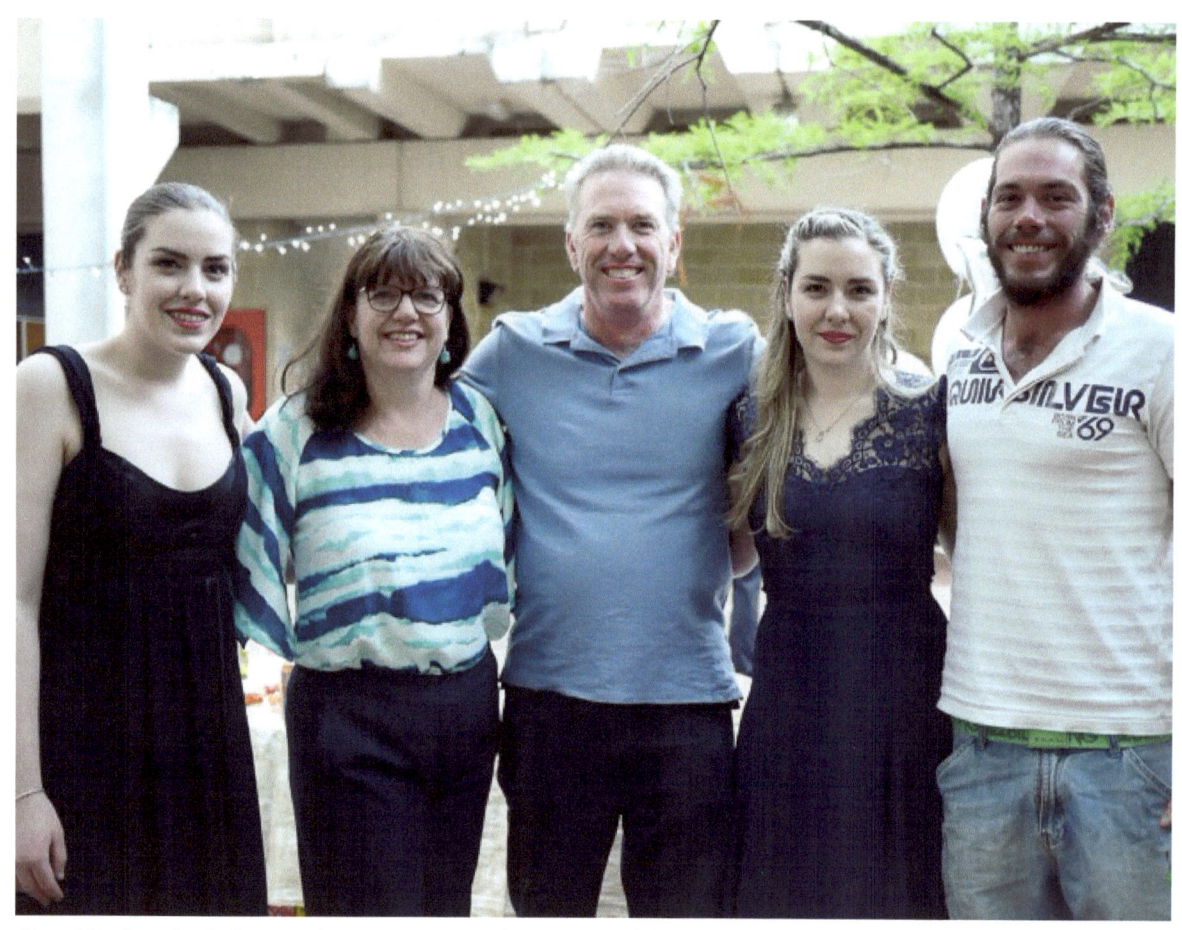

Gerald's family, left to right: Monique, Alison, Gerald, Genevieve and Brayden

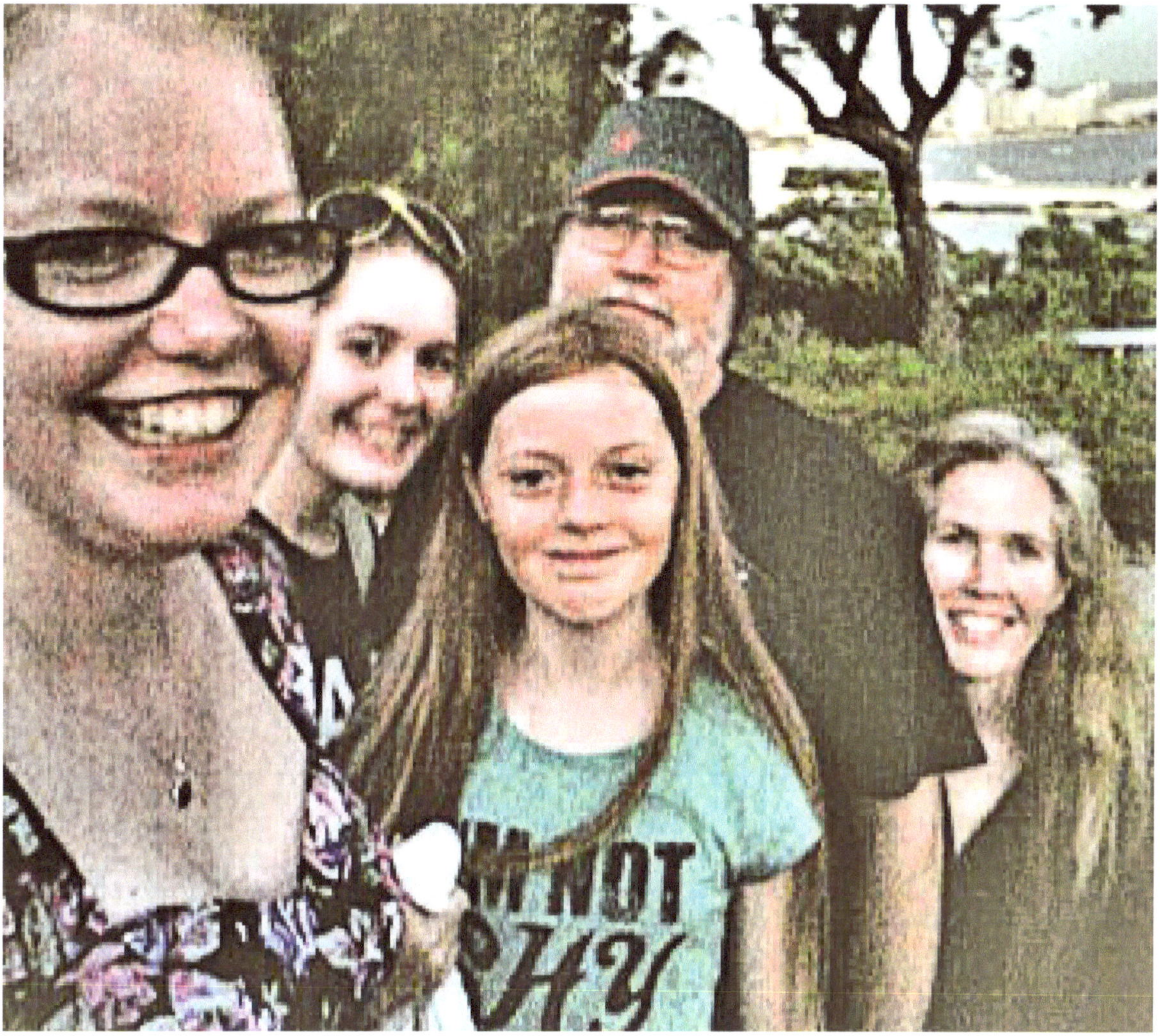

Wendy's family, left to right: Kristy-Lee, Jessie, Breanna, Noel and Wendy

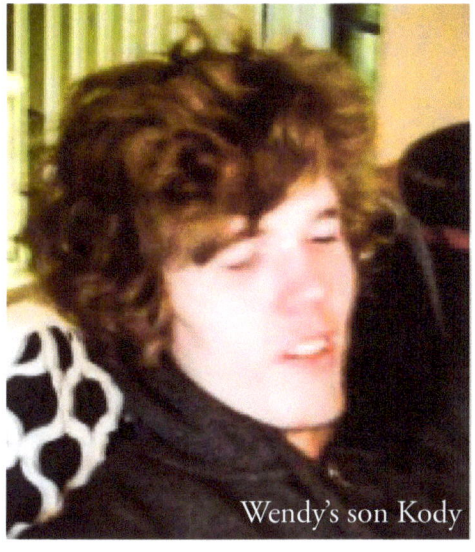

Wendy's son Kody

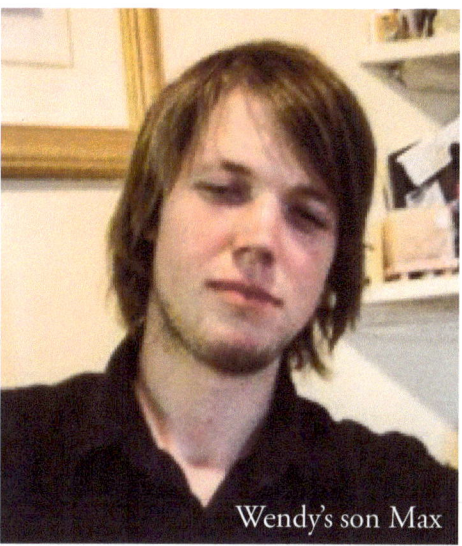

Wendy's son Max

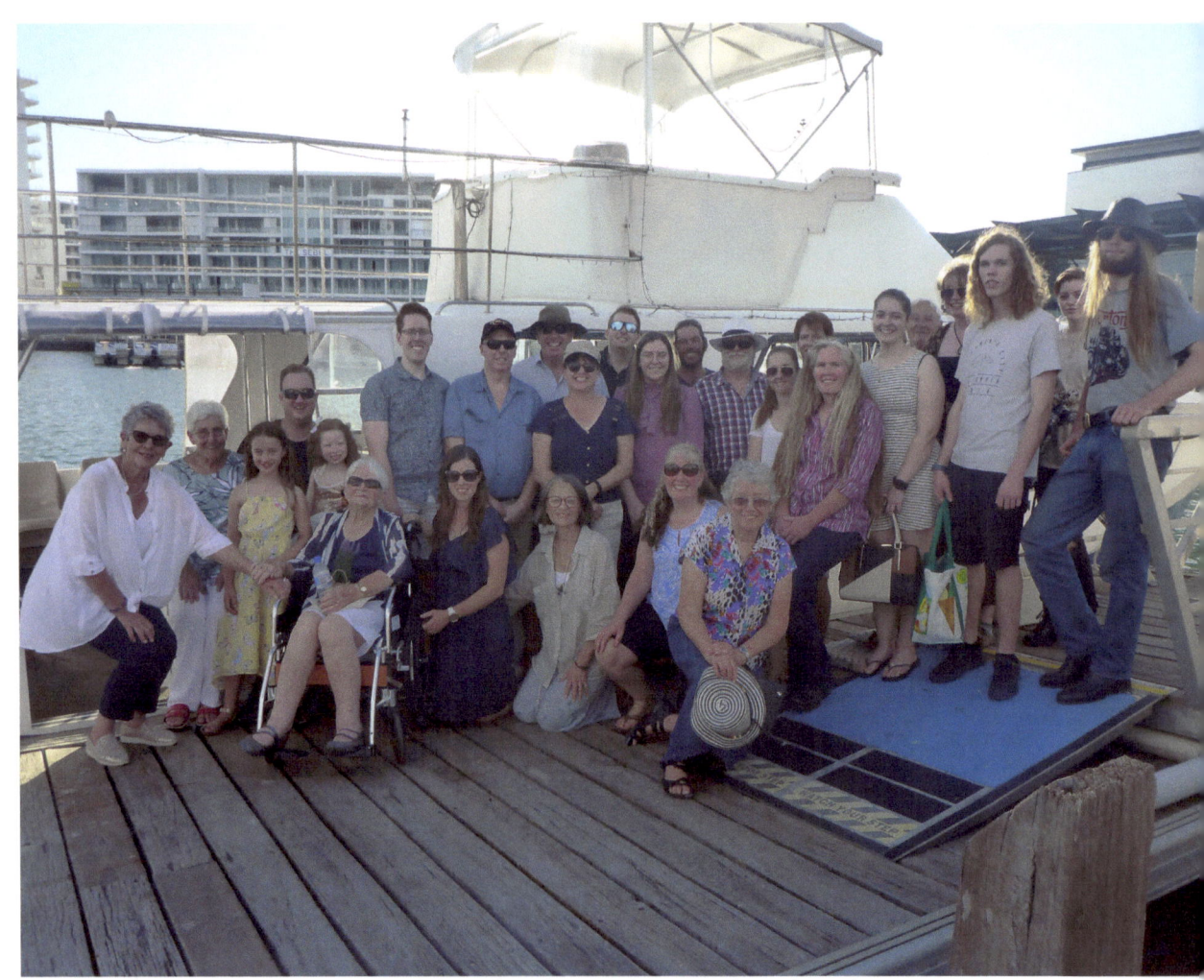
2021, Me with my children and their families, and some of my friends

To my beautiful granddaughter, you have done such a fantastic job putting my script and photos together into such a nice book! Thank you so much Monique!!

www.ingramcontent.com/pod-product-compliance
Lightning Source LLC
Chambersburg PA
CBHW041412160426
42811CB00107B/1778